8-99

A014063476

TAKING CO

CW01401545

Taking control

A *new approach to living with arthritis*

Margaret Gore

ALLEN & UNWIN

Dedication

*To Lisby, Iain and Thursday, without whom I would not
have been able to maintain my sense of humour*

First published in 1998
Allen & Unwin
9 Atchison Street, St Leonards NSW 2065 Australia
Phone: (61 2) 9901 4088
Fax: (61 2) 9906 2218
E-mail: frontdesk@allen-unwin.com.au
Web: http://www.allen-unwin.com.au

National Library of Australia
Cataloguing-in-Publication entry:

Gore, Margaret, 1946– .
    Taking control: a new approach to living with arthritis.

    ISBN 1 86448 691 0.

    1. Arthritis—Popular works. 2. Arthritis—Treatment—Popular works
    I. Title.

616.72203

Set in 11.5/13.5 pt Garamond by DOCUPRO, Sydney
Printed and bound by McPhersons Printing Group, Australia

10 9 8 7 6 5 4 3 2 1

Contents

Part 2 Understanding arthritis

Acknowledgements

The author would like to thank the following people and organisations for their invaluable help in the production of this book: The Arthritis Foundation of Australia; The Arthritis Foundation of NSW; Dr Peter Brooks, Professor of Medicine, University of NSW; St Vincent's Hospital; The Commonwealth Department of Health; The Independent Living Centre of NSW; The Australasian College of Natural Therapies; Dr Sue Carruthers. I would also like to thank C.M. Smeeton for his illustrations.

The medical information provided in this book is for educational purposes only. The information provided is not a substitute for a professional medical opinion. If you have any concerns about your or your family's health, please see your doctor for treatment and advice.

Introduction

In 1995 I achieved a long-held dream of buying some land to build a home and establish an organic herb farm. The same month that I moved onto the property I was diagnosed with osteoarthritis in my knees and hands and told that I could no longer do any heavy gardening work, let alone pursue an agricultural lifestyle. I was devastated, not only by the diagnosis of arthritis, which I never suspected could happen at my age—I was only in my forties—but also by the news that I was no longer physically capable of realising a goal I had been striving for, for twenty years. I went into a tailspin of depression and experienced all the classic symptoms of shock, denial, resentment and fear, that I later discovered were common reactions to this diagnosis.

Feeling lost and confused about my situation I went in search of information about the disease—I wanted to find something to give me hope, encouragement, practical advice and an understanding of what I was feeling. When the shelves of my local library and bookstore failed to give me what I was looking for, my journalistic training asserted itself and I started researching the subject in detail.

What I learned was that arthritis affects a great many people—not only those diagnosed with the disease but also their family and friends. There are, in fact, over 150 forms of arthritis and nearly two million Australians suffer from it in some way. It can affect people of all ages. Two out of every three people with the disease are under the age of 65, and many of these are young children.

In this book I have focused on the types of arthritis that affect the most people: the degenerative (osteoarthritis) and inflammatory (rheumatoid arthritis) forms; crystal deposition disease (gout); and juvenile arthritis. Although symptoms and treatment might vary slightly for the lesser known forms of arthritis, the general principles of managing the illness outlined here apply equally well for all arthritis sufferers.

Arthritis is a term for inflammation of one or more joints and humans have suffered from it ever since prehistoric days, as evidenced by the skeletal remains of prehistoric man. Once arthritis was feared as a painful, crippling disease which often caused people to age before their time; today, while a cure has yet to be found, there are many new and effective ways to manage this condition. Greater understanding of the disease, new pharmaceutical developments and surgical procedures, advances in prostheses, physiotherapy and occupational therapy, mean that for most sufferers, symptoms can be minimised, pain relieved, joints replaced if necessary and quality of life maintained.

Arthritis affects everyone differently—physically, mentally and emotionally. For some people, it's a mild condition which doesn't interfere with their daily lives; other people face debilitating pain, fatigue and depression. Whether your arthritis is acute or chronic, knowledge is a powerful weapon in the fight to minimise pain and joint damage and maximise your health and well-being.

All forms of arthritis need accurate diagnosis and appropriate treatment. Whatever form of arthritis you're suffering from, the key to managing the disease is education. The more you learn about your arthritis the more you'll be able to make positive decisions and follow a course of treatment that is right for you.

In the first half of this book I look at what it's like for you and your family to live with arthritis—the practical and emotional aspects of living with the disease from day-to-day.

The second half of the book is devoted to a down-to-earth A–Z Guide to help fill in any gaps in your understanding of the cause, effect and treatment of your arthritis. I also look at alternative and complementary therapies to help maximise your health care, enhance your sense of well-being and improve your quality of life.

I found that taking practical steps to manage my arthritis gave me a sense of being in control and removed that dreadful feeling of being a 'victim' of the disease.

So take heart! If your arthritis has left you in pain, depressed and vulnerable, you can change all that. You can take charge of the condition, and turn it around so that it has minimum effects on your quality of life. As I have found, being diagnosed with arthritis isn't the end of the world. As the old saying goes, 'one door closes, another one opens'— and it's perfectly true of living with arthritis. Your life doesn't have to stop just because you have it. You may not be able to do all the things you used to do, but this can be an opportunity to take up new and exciting interests. Accepting arthritis as a challenge can give you a new purpose in life; looking after your diet and getting more exercise can actually make you feel better than you have in years. You may have to adjust your lifestyle a little but that doesn't have to lessen your quality of life. It can simply be a matter of doing things differently.

I hope you find this book helpful in achieving better health and the personal goals in your life. By the way, the herb farm is coming along nicely now!

Best wishes,
Margaret Gore

Part 1

Take charge of your arthritis

1

Coming to terms
with arthritis

Being diagnosed with arthritis comes as quite a shock, as I found out. After weeks of rest and physiotherapy for a painful, stiff knee, my doctor sent me to see an orthopaedic surgeon. His diagnosis was that there was probably a torn piece of cartilage floating around in my knee irritating the synovium, thus causing the inflammation, swelling and pain. An arthroscopy would fix it up in no time! When the surgeon came to see me in the recovery ward he told me that the situation was much worse than he thought and that my knee showed advanced osteoarthritis, with the cartilage worn so thin that raw bone was exposed in some areas. I was to go home, rest and see him in a week.

I was stunned. What did this mean? What would happen to me if I had a worn-out knee? Did this mean I was going to be crippled? I spent the week feeling depressed and with a million questions rattling around my brain. Things didn't improve at my next appointment as the surgeon told me that I was too young to have a knee replacement. Drug therapy could keep the pain under control, but I was to avoid any activity which could put strain on my knee joint, such as sports like tennis, or daily activities like carrying shopping, kneeling, or any type of heavy gardening work. As I was about to fulfil my lifelong dream of becoming a farmer, this came as a particularly heavy blow. I was simply given a prescription for a non-steroidal anti-inflammatory drug and told to come back in six weeks. I stumbled into the street in tears. I felt overwhelmed by a mixture of emotions—extremely vulnerable; angry that my body had let me down; frustrated that modern medicine couldn't fix the problem; aged before my time; and frightened about what this would mean for my future.

Arthritis is not one of those 'pale and interesting' diseases that arouses much sympathy. It's more likely to evoke responses like, 'What is she going on about? It's only arthritis after all.' I've learned that non-sufferers view it as no great problem, just something you should 'grin and bear'. So on top of all the other emotions, I began to feel isolated. I felt myself slipping into deep depression and I knew I had to do something about it. I realised that I had to educate myself about my condition if I was going to get on top of it. In doing so, I've learned about the other forms of arthritis and realised that even though I had now been diagnosed with arthritis in my hands as well, my problems did not compare with what other sufferers had to deal with.

I also discovered that by taking a pro-active approach, you can overcome a great many of the associated problems. First, because learning everything you can about your illness makes you feel in control of the situation rather than vulnerable to it. Second, because you're taking positive steps to overcome symptoms, improve your overall health and learn about relaxation and stress control, your sense of well-being increases, people respond more positively to you, and this in turn lifts your outlook on life.

COMMON REACTIONS TO A DIAGNOSIS OF ARTHRITIS

- *denial* 'I haven't got it, they must be wrong.'
- *complacency* 'They'll find a cure, so I don't have to worry.'
- *negativity* 'My life is over, there is nothing I can do!'
- *self-pity* 'Why me?'
- *vulnerability* 'What is going to happen to me?'

- *anger* 'I've things I want to do in my life!'
- *grief* 'I never did go trekking in the Himalayas.'
- *depression* 'I used to be able to do so much!'

As I learned, these are perfectly normal reactions to a diagnosis of arthritis and part of the recognised 'acceptance period' that most people go through when faced with a degenerative disease. It's important to let yourself feel things such as grief because your life has changed, but try not to become consumed by self-pity which is not only destructive to you but can erode the sympathy and support you need from your family and friends. Keep in mind that arthritis is not a life-threatening illness and that medical, surgical and physical treatment can reduce symptoms, prevent disability and maintain your quality of life well into old age.

This is a delicate period emotionally and how you react now can make a great deal of difference to your well-being, as the following stories show.

Ben was a young computer programmer in his late twenties who was making a name for himself in the information technology industry. Dedicated and hardworking, he had put his increasingly stiff back down to long hours sitting at his computer. He consulted a chiropractor, then an osteopath to see if they could loosen up his spine and though he felt the treatment gave him temporary relief the overall problem gradually became worse.

Eventually he consulted his doctor. After blood tests and x-rays, Ben was diagnosed with ankylosing spondylitis, a form of arthritis affecting the joints between the vertebrae of the lower spine and the sacroiliac joints in the pelvis. Ankylosing spondylitis can lead to permanent stiffness in, and curvature of, the spine. Ben was devastated. To him, arthritis was an old man's disease and he later admitted that his mind shut out what the doctor was telling him.

The diagnosis sent him into a spiral of anger, depression and fear. At first he took the medication his doctor prescribed, but when it started to give him indigestion he stopped. He started taking time off work and lying in bed all day. His back was getting stiffer and more painful. He dropped his friends as he didn't want them to see him in this state and he alienated his family with his anger and moods. In a few months Ben was hardly able to get out of bed, convinced that he was crippled for life.

Ben was finally rescued from his mental and physical distress by a family friend who was a physiotherapist. She explained the disease to him in such a way that he actually listened to her. He went back to the doctor and his medication was changed to one he could tolerate well, and the physiotherapist designed a program of gentle manipulation and exercise that started loosening his spine. She also encouraged Ben to take up swimming and learn how to maintain good posture and joint care. Within months he was back at work, had resumed a social life, and felt fitter and more limber than he had in years.

Julie was married with three children and a part-time job. When she didn't recover from what she thought was a bad bout of 'flu, she went to her doctor and was diagnosed with rheumatoid arthritis. Like Ben, she was devastated, as the disease left her exhausted and in pain to the point where she could neither work nor look after her family. However, unlike Ben, she was determined to beat it. Even in her weakened state she learned all she could about her arthritis, and worked with her doctor, physiotherapist, and family to design a program which would keep her symptoms under control, boost her general health, and keep daily life not only manageable but enjoyable too.

Although Julie could never predict how she was going to feel from day to day, or week to week, she felt in control of her situation, well supported by her family and health team and able to lead a reasonably normal life.

You can see why it's important to come to terms with your arthritis—accept that you have it, and treat it as a challenge—because your approach can have a vast impact on your quality of life. By taking control of the situation and fostering a positive attitude, you'll go a long way to making yourself, and those around you, feel better; you'll recognise that it isn't the end of the world and that life—and a good one at that—goes on. Early medical intervention, combined with good physical therapy and a sound pain management plan, has often led an arthritis sufferer to a better, more enjoyable life than they had before.

UNDERSTANDING ARTHRITIS

One of the best ways of taking charge of this disease is to learn as much as you can about it. Make a list of questions you would like your doctor to answer. Writing your questions down is helpful because the atmosphere in a doctor's rooms can often make you forget what you want to ask. Don't be shy about wanting to know more. Some doctors need lots of prompting to explain things thoroughly. What follows is a general outline of the most common types of arthritis. There is more detailed information in the 'A–Z guide to arthritis' (page 133).

Most forms of arthritis involve inflammation, pain and swelling in one or more joints. To understand how the various forms of arthritis develop, it's important to know how a normal joint works. A joint is the junction of two or more bones. There are different types of joints in the body—some are fixed, such as those in the skull; some allow a small amount of movement as in the vertebrae of the

A normal joint

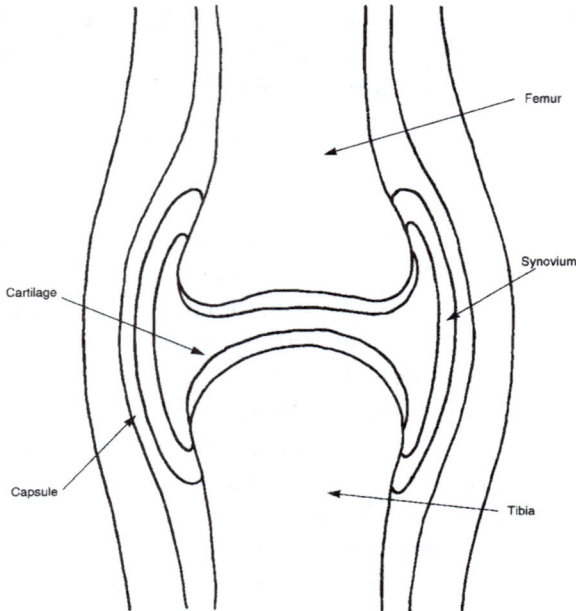

Femur

Synovium

Cartilage

Capsule

Tibia

spine; while others are designed to allow a large range of motion such as the hips, knees and elbows. It's usually the mobile joints that are affected by arthritis.

The ends of the bones in these joints are covered by a smooth, tough material called cartilage which acts as a shock absorber and allows the joint to move easily. The joint is enclosed in a strong fibrous capsule lined by a membrane called the synovium, which produces a lubricating fluid. This synovial fluid not only allows the joint to move smoothly but nourishes the cartilage and removes any waste products from the area.

If you are diagnosed with **osteoarthritis** it will be in a synovial joint, usually a weight-bearing joint such as the knee, hip, lower back and neck, but it can also be a shoulder, thumb, finger or big toe. Osteoarthritis can affect people to differing degrees. Some people only have mild or occasional aches, while others suffer stiffness, swelling and severe pain which persists even when resting. Commonly known as the 'wear and tear' disease, the actual cause of osteoarthritis is unknown, although it is thought to occur when cellular changes within the joint cause the cartilage to thin, become brittle, then flake off. These changes cause the joint to become stiff, swollen and painful. As the condition persists, the cartilage erodes to the point where raw bone is exposed, and over time bony spurs called osteophytes grow out from the margins of the bone causing the joint to become deformed.

Treatment is based on medication and physical therapy and there is plenty you can do to slow the degenerative process, relieve stiffness, swelling and pain, and increase your mobility, overall health and fitness (see 'A–Z guide to arthritis' page 133).

Although the symptoms may appear to be similar, **rheumatoid arthritis** is quite distinct from osteoarthritis. Rheumatoid arthritis is an autoimmune disease in which pain and swelling occurs in previously healthy joints, caused by some unknown factor. It's an unpredictable disease which can strike suddenly or develop gradually; it can be confined to a single episode, or experienced as a prolonged series of attacks, and bouts of illness or remission occur for no apparent reason. Symptoms, which include aching, swollen and/or stiff joints, fever, fatigue and insomnia, can vary from person to person with some patients experiencing only minor aches and pains, while others are totally debilitated by the disease. The cause of rheumatoid arthritis has yet to be discovered, but it's thought to occur when the immune system malfunctions. As yet medical science has found no cure, however, medication and physical therapy can contain the disease and ensure your quality of life is maintained.

People with **gout** have been the butt of jokes for centuries, but for sufferers it's no laughing matter, as the pain can be excruciating. One of the most common types of arthritis, gout occurs in ten times as many men as women. Normally only one joint is affected, usually the big toe, but it can also occur in the ankle, knee, elbow, wrist or hand.

Onset can be sudden with the joint rapidly swelling, becoming red and painful, and pain increasing over the next one or two days.

Gout is caused by uric acid crystals precipitating out of the blood stream into the joint spaces and surrounding tissue, which irritate the synovium, and trigger the inflammatory process which produces the symptoms (see 'A–Z guide' page 133).

One form of arthritis which affects people in their early adulthood is **systemic lupus erythematosus (SLE)**, a chronic inflammatory disease affecting not only joints but other body tissues and organs. Like rheumatoid arthritis, SLE (often called lupus) is an autoimmune disease which causes inflammation and debilitating symptoms including fever, weakness, fatigue, weight loss, rashes, morning stiffness and joint pain, aching muscles, swollen glands, loss of appetite, hair loss, nausea and vomiting. As yet no cause or cure has been identified. Patients are subject to flare-ups and remissions as with other inflammatory arthritic conditions and it is treated in much the same way as rheumatoid arthritis (see 'A–Z guide' page 133).

Ankylosing spondylitis is seen in almost one in a hundred people, and affects more men than women, often when they are in their twenties and thirties. It presents as inflammation of the joints in the spine and causes stiffness and eventually rigidity of the back. First signs of ankylosing spondylitis are stiffness in the hips and lower back, especially first thing in the morning. Other symptoms include decreased mobility and pain in the hips, knees, heels, ankles and chest. No cure has yet been found, so treatment relies on managing the condition with medication, physical therapy, and daily exercise (see 'A–Z guide' page 133).

Sometimes arthritis is hard to diagnose and a number of conditions come under the heading of **seronegative arthritis**. These present with the symptoms of rheumatoid arthritis in a number of joints, but show no sign of the rheumatoid marker when blood tests are taken. This form of arthritis can be connected with Crohn's disease (an inflammatory disorder of the intestines), autoimmune diseases, and skin conditions such as psoriasis. Even though the form of the arthritis can't be pinpointed, its symptoms are very real with stiffness, pain and swelling in the joints. It's treated in a similar way to rheumatoid arthritis, which is usually successful in managing the condition.

Understanding the medical side of the illness is only part of the solution. It's also important to learn how to manage your illness on a day-to-day basis and I discuss this in more detail in Chapter 2. One organisation which can help you learn to manage your disease is the Arthritis Foundation of Australia. It has over 70 branches around the country and offers support in a variety of ways:

- *education seminars* Help you acquire the knowledge and skill to manage your arthritis effectively. Courses are usually held in local community centres or hospitals and last for about two hours a week for six weeks.
- *hydrotherapy* Water exercise classes conducted by trained volunteers in specially heated pools. Warm water exercise brings pain relief, combined with long lasting improvements in joint mobility and muscle strength.
- *discussion groups* You can meet fellow sufferers and be able to discuss arthritis and other topics such as coping with household tasks, gardening, handicrafts and cooking, etc.
- *walking groups* These groups conduct regular gentle exercise and walking programs. Joining one of these groups can encourage you to actually take regular exercise by setting a weekly time and place for the activity and providing companionship as well.

For all these activities and more, contact your nearest Arthritis Foundation branch. See 'Where to go for help and further information', page 175.

2

Your management plan and quality of life

One of the most important factors in taking charge of your arthritis is to develop an effective management plan and support team. A management plan involves taking medication, having physical therapy, eating well, doing regular gentle exercise, practising relaxation techniques and adopting a positive outlook on life. Your support team includes:

- your family and friends for practical help and encouragement as well as love and affection
- your doctor to prescribe medication, check side effects, advise on other treatment, and monitor your overall health
- a physiotherapist to mobilise your joints, administer therapy to reduce symptoms and advise on appropriate exercise to maintain your mobility
- a podiatrist to advise on correct footwear and the use of orthoses and prostheses to correct any mechanical problems in your feet, legs or back
- a dietitian to help you work out an eating plan to help you lose weight if you need to and maximise nutrition and health
- your hairdresser to give you a style that is both flattering and easy to care for if your hands are affected by arthritis.

Family support is crucial and I discuss the implications for family and friends of arthritis sufferers in Chapter 11. It's important that they read that chapter, if not the whole book, so you can discuss how you all feel about your illness, any problems that you might be experiencing, and work out a management plan that will suit everybody's needs. Involving everyone in this way makes them feel included, provides emotional strength for you and promotes better communication and understanding in the family as a whole.

GETTING THE BEST FROM YOUR DOCTOR

The next most important factor in staying on top of arthritis is your relationship with your doctor and specialist. Some doctors may seem aloof and uncommunicative, but if you take an active interest in learning about your arthritis and give the treatment they suggest a fair go, it can improve your doctor/patient relationship tremendously. Most doctors actually like *working with* their patients to overcome problems, rather than simply *dictating* to them. So ask questions, and report any changes in the way you feel—and you'll probably find your doctor will be encouraged, gain greater satisfaction from your progress, and feel that they are actually doing some good.

Sometimes patients with arthritis project their anger, frustration and fear onto their doctor. They want the doctor to 'fix' the problem, and when they can't (because there isn't a cure) the patient becomes difficult and resists the doctor's recommendations.

Sophie was a classic case of this. In her sixties, she was diagnosed with osteoarthritis in both knees. Busily involved with charitable organisations, she was a leading light in her community. The problem with her knees was slowing her up and she wanted something done about it and fast. Her doctor referred her to a specialist who prescribed anti-inflammatories, exercise and a weight loss program. Sophie was furious because she felt she was being blamed for causing the illness by being overweight. She expected more of modern medicine than being told to 'take a few pills and go for a walk' as she saw it. She went back to her doctor demanding a second opinion. She ended up seeing several specialists with the same result.

By this time, Sophie was in a state of barely suppressed rage, her condition seemed to have worsened and she was making life hell for herself and all around her. It got to the point where her doctor dreaded to see her name in his appointment book. Sophie's pent up emotions came to a head one day when she collapsed in uncontrollable tears in the middle of a supermarket. Finally, she was persuaded to join an education program sponsored by the Arthritis Foundation which helped her come to terms with the disease. She started following the recommended treatment program and began to feel better. She lost weight and began exercising. Soon she felt younger than she had in years.

Sophie's case was an extreme example, but many patients feel resentment towards their doctor if no 'quick medical fix' is available. So it's important to keep in mind that your doctors will do everything they can to help you—that's what they're there for—but doctors are only human. Ask yourself which you would rather deal with—a pleasant cooperative patient or a difficult, resentful one? This doesn't mean you should accept treatment you're not sure of or happy with, but discussing your concerns with the doctor, rather than challenging their recommendation, will elicit a far more positive outcome for you. Here are some strategies that may help.

• Learn as much as you can about treatment for your form

of arthritis, any new developments and the outlook for the future.

- Ask your doctor, or other health workers, to explain the treatment they are recommending. If you don't understand the first time, ask them to explain it again more simply. Sometimes doctors forget that we don't all have medical degrees!
- Make a commitment to stick with any recommended management plan—at least for a period of time—to see if the results are beneficial.
- Take your medication exactly the way they are prescribed.
- Report any symptoms or side effects to your doctor—don't just put up with them silently or, worse still, stop taking the medication.

Between visits to your doctor

While taking your medication and following your management plan, it's a good idea to keep a health diary and write down when you're feeling well or unwell. Note any other symptoms and the days when you feel more pain or fatigue. See if there is a pattern to this. If symptoms persist, make a note to mention them to your doctor at your next appointment. Also, whenever you think of something you'd like to ask your doctor, make a note of it. Before you go to your next appointment, write a short summarised progress report and take it with you so that when your doctor asks you how you are and if the medications are helping, you can give her accurate information.

If you have a number of questions and a lot you want to discuss with your doctor, it's helpful if you explain this to the receptionist so that you can be booked in for a longer appointment.

At the appointment

Take your health diary with you, so you can answer questions accurately. Ask your own questions and after the consultation, take a few minutes in the waiting room to make some notes of what has been said. By the time you get home you may not be able to recall the information as clearly as immediately after the visit.

Don't be afraid to admit your fears

If you're worried about the side effects of drugs or the long-term outlook for your health, don't be afraid to tell your doctor for fear of appearing silly or neurotic. By talking about your concerns, your doctor can allay your fears and sort out any problems you may be having. This is true for all patients, not just those suffering from arthritis. When any treatment is prescribed, here are some questions everyone should ask their doctor.

- What effect will it have on the disease?
- What, if any, are the side effects?
- What will happen if you don't have this treatment?
- How much will it cost?

It's important to ask 'What effect will it have on the disease?' so you know what improvements to expect, and how to gauge the effectiveness of the treatment.

The questions about side effects and not having the treatment go together because there may be a risk of mild side effects from certain treatments, but there may be far worse consequences from not having the treatment.

How much it will cost is important because you should know up-front what costs you are liable for, whether your health insurance or Medicare will cover the cost, whether there is a gap you will have to pay and whether there is a generic version of any medication which is prescribed. Often the generic version is just as effective but costs much less than a brand name.

MEDICATIONS

While there are no miracle cures for arthritis, modern medicine can do a great deal to control most forms and certainly give the majority of people relief from symptoms.

So if you are diagnosed with any form of arthritis, don't leave the condition untreated—lack of proper therapy will only lead to joint damage, loss of mobility and ultimately increased pain. Many people worry about taking long-term medication for fear of side effects. The truth is that most people *don't* suffer adverse reactions to their medication and if they do, these are usually mild and go away once the medication or dosage is changed. It's important to realise that the long-term effects of arthritis far outweigh any temporary side effects that drug therapy *might* cause.

For example, if you have been diagnosed with rheumatoid arthritis, it may be recommended that you take disease-modifying anti-rheumatic drugs—these may cause some side effects which careful monitoring can detect and control. Taking these drugs will relieve your symptoms and minimise joint, cartilage and bone damage. *Not* taking the drugs can lead to a rapid deterioration in your condition, because joints are permanently damaged by rheumatoid arthritis within six to twelve months from the onset of the disease. So the consequences of not taking the drugs far outweigh the possible temporary side effects of taking them.

Onset of some forms of arthritis, notably rheumatoid arthritis and gout, should be treated as a medical emergency. If you've been diagnosed as only having had the disease for six months or so, then aggressive drug therapy could rid you of it. Another reason for seeking early treatment is that if you put off being treated, your condition will be much harder to control.

Learn as much as you can about the different drugs which may be prescribed, what they are prescribed for, how they work, and what the outcome should be. The three main purposes of arthritis medication are to:

- relieve pain
- reduce inflammation
- slow the progress of the disease.

Some drugs are for immediate symptom relief, such as the analgesics and non-steroidal anti-inflammatory drugs

(NSAIDs) while others, such as the disease-modifying anti-rheumatic drugs, have long-term benefits.

It's also important to understand why a particular drug is being prescribed for you and to know of any side effects you should watch out for. Make sure you understand how and when it should be taken and any possible interaction with other medications you might be taking, both prescribed and over-the-counter. Drugs used in the treatment of arthritis include:

- analgesics
- non-steroidal anti-inflammatory drugs (NSAIDs)
- specific gout drugs
- corticosteroids
- disease-modifying or slow-acting anti-rheumatic drugs (DMARDs or SAARDs).

DON'T MIX AND MATCH YOUR HEALTH CARE

To get the best outcome from any course of treatment, it's important to give it a 'fair go' to prove its efficacy in treating your disease. In most cases this takes time—sometimes weeks, maybe even months—and you may be tempted to give up or switch to something else. However, even though progress may seem slow, it's best if you continue for the recommended time. If there is no real improvement at the end of that time, then a different treatment can be tried.

What's not good is to mix and match your treatment, tempting though it may be to do so. Try to resist the 'surefire-cures' suggested by colleagues or magazine articles which claim miraculous results in no time at all.

Susie was a young mother in her early thirties diagnosed with rheumatoid arthritis. She first consulted her doctor, who outlined the various medications that could be used to treat her condition.

She took the prescribed drugs for a while, but stopped them when she read an article about the curative powers of evening primrose oil. A few weeks later, with her symptoms no better, she switched to ginger tablets and a yeast-free diet, recommended by her local health food shop owner. Finally after several months, she returned to her doctor claiming to be no better but didn't admit she'd changed her treatment.

Now I'm not saying Susie shouldn't have considered natural therapies to treat her illness, but it would have been wise to talk to her doctor first or consult a properly qualified herbalist or naturopath who was a member of the National Herbalists Association of Australia, the Australian Natural Therapists Association or the Australian Traditional Medicine Society. Following the orthodox or alternative medical route is really a question for you to decide but, whichever you choose, make sure to learn as much as you can about the treatment each offers, then make a commitment to following the one you choose. This way you'll have the best chance for a positive outcome.

UNPROVEN REMEDIES

Many doctors working with arthritis patients are concerned about the 'unproven remedies' recommended by alternative therapists, folk medicine, or advertisements in newspapers and magazines. These fall into three categories: the harmless, the harmful and the 'jury's still out'. The harmless include apple cider vinegar, garlic and honey, ginger, crystal therapy, copper bracelets; the harmful include snake venom, mega doses of vitamins and minerals, and purchased remedies with hidden ingredients such as steroids; the jury is still out on many of the herbal remedies, food allergies, biofeedback and laser therapies.

Many people turn to alternative treatment because they feel that conventional medicine has failed them in some way. I don't have a closed mind about complementary medicine. However, it's important to know that delaying medical treatment, especially for conditions like rheumatoid arthritis and lupus (SLE), can lead to greater joint damage, making the disease more intractable and harder to treat. So it's essential to consider your options carefully before choosing which route to take.

Be wary of any remedy which:

- · claims to be based on a secret formula
- claims to work for all forms of arthritis
- uses case histories and testimonials as proof of efficacy
- cites only one study
- cites a study without a control group
- doesn't list its ingredient
- doesn't warn about any side effects.

DIET

There is much debate about the effects of diet on various forms of arthritis. What is known is that:

- Diet plays an important role in the management of gout, with sufferers advised to avoid alcohol and foods such as anchovies, poultry, pulses, sardines and yeast products, which contain purine, a substance which can raise uric acid levels in the blood stream.
- Losing weight, for those who are over their height-to-weight ratio, can reduce stress on joints and help slow down the rate of degeneration and improve mobility for those suffering from osteoarthritis.
- Omega-3 fatty acids found in foods like oily fish such

as tuna, sardines, salmon, etc., have anti-inflammatory effects, so including fish two or three times a week may help reduce inflammation in joints.
- Overall health can be improved by adopting a low-fat, high-fibre, well-balanced diet (for more information see Chapter 9).

EXERCISE

Exercise is an important element in the treatment of arthritis to maintain mobility, reduce stress and fatigue, and improve overall well-being. By exercise I mean not just walking, swimming, cycling, etc., but also daily stretching and 'range-of-motion exercises' to keep you supple, maintain good circulation, muscle tone, weight control and improve sleep. Here, your physiotherapist is your best ally. Physiotherapists can not only mobilise stiff joints and provide treatment to relieve pain, but can also help you work out an exercise program that suits you and supply you with a series of daily stretches to keep you as flexible as possible.

Adding exercise to your daily management plan can bring vast improvements to your overall health, as well as relieving arthritis symptoms. Even doing a few stretches before you get out of bed in the morning, or after a warm shower, can make all the difference to how you feel for the rest of the day (see Chapter 8). Exercising in warm water (hydrotherapy) also allows you to perform range-of-motion exercises while your body weight is supported by water. Under the expert eye of a trained instructor, hydrotherapy classes can reduce swelling and make your muscles stronger, your joints more supple and less painful. Exercise in general has very positive benefits including:

- decreasing pain
- keeping joints mobile
- increasing muscle strength
- strengthening bones and ligaments
- preventing joint deformities
- providing nourishment to the joints

- increasing general health and fitness
- maintaining and increasing your ability to perform daily tasks.

Suitable exercise includes swimming, walking, cycling, gentle stretch classes, yoga, Tai Chi and gentle aquarobics (see Chapter 8 for more details).

THE REST AND EXERCISE BALANCE

One crucial aspect of managing this disease is to learn to balance rest and exercise. It's vital to keep your affected joint/s flexible to prevent stiffness and immobility, however if they're inflamed, it's just as important to rest them. Be sensible in your approach to this. Soldiering on when you're in pain is only going to make matters worse, but avoiding exercise when you are perfectly capable of doing it misses an opportunity to keep your joints mobile. It's a fine balance and only you can know which is appropriate at any one time.

When the disease is in its more active phase, rest your joints to reduce inflammation and pain, but this doesn't necessarily mean bed rest—it can also mean wearing a splint, using crutches or walking sticks, or doing actions in a different way. For instance, if your fingers are sore but you must use your hands, avoid any kind of wrenching or twisting movements, and when standing, walking or carrying items try to distribute the weight evenly over several joints.

Try to plan your day so that active periods are followed by rest. For instance, cleaning and tidying could be followed by some seated activity such as computer work or writing letters.

EQUIPMENT THAT CAN HELP

Using special gadgets and equipment for everyday activities can also make a big difference to easing symptoms and saving joints from further wear and tear. For example, kitchen equipment for removing jar lids, or knives with specially adapted handles, can prevent your hands from being strained during the simple preparation of a meal (see Chapter 7).

SURGERY

If, however, your joint is so badly deformed or painful that your quality of life is being severely affected, then surgery may be called for. This could involve joint replacement (arthroplasty) or immobilisation (arthrodesis). Joints can be replaced in the hip, knee, finger, shoulder and elbow, although hip and knee joint replacement operations are the most common. Immobilisation is performed to reduce pain and stabilise joints such as in the fingers or disc joints in the spine (see 'A–Z guide to arthritis' page 133).

QUALITY OF LIFE

It's now well documented that people who choose to look on the bright side of life suffer less fatigue, sleep better, have a stronger immune system and a reduced perception of pain than people with a negative outlook.

Here are some things to try to do:

- Cultivate a positive attitude to life—think of the glass being half-full, rather than half-empty. Read self-help books on the power of positive thinking or attend classes which can help you take a more optimistic outlook on life.
- Be as healthy as you possibly can—physically, mentally and emotionally. Eat a healthy diet, include some exercise in your day, try to get enough sleep; include stimulating activities in your life such as going to movies, plays or concerts, visit art galleries and museums, listen to beautiful music, read good books, enjoy social gatherings.
- Be as independent as possible—this doesn't mean stubbornly refusing all help. Take a sensible approach, stand on your own two feet where you can, but don't be afraid to ask for help if you need it.
- Live for today—this is something we should all do.

Sometimes we spend so much time worrying about what 'might' happen in the future that we miss the enjoyable things that are occurring right now.

- Enjoy life—easy to say, but not always easy to do, especially if you have to live with chronic pain. However, take time in every day to appreciate the good things, no matter how simple, that exist in your life—the beauty of a rose in your garden, the pattern of clouds in the sky, a piece of inspirational music, the company of someone you love. Stop, feel and appreciate the moment—it will make you feel a lot better about life.

Having quality of life involves taking your medication, having physical therapy, eating well, doing regular gentle exercise, practising relaxation techniques and adopting a positive outlook on life.

3

Overcoming pain

One of the most difficult aspects of living with arthritis is dealing with pain. As we all feel pain differently, no one solution works for everyone. Some people have a high tolerance of pain, while others have a very low pain threshold; some experience acute pain which lasts only during a 'flare-up', while others suffer persistent, gnawing agony. Both types can lead to stress and depression which in turn makes the perception of pain more acute.

WHAT IS PAIN?

Pain is an unpleasant sensation which can range from mild discomfort to intolerable agony. It is created by special sensory nerves connected to the thalamus in the brain and is the body's way of telling us that something is wrong—that we have sustained an injury, or that repeating an action will lead to injury, or that infection is present. It's a way of getting us to do something about it.

Pain from arthritis has several causes:

- *inflammation* present in all forms of arthritis to a greater or lesser extent. It's responsible for the swelling, redness, warmth and stiffness in the joint

25

- *joint damage* caused by erosion of the joint tissues
- *muscle tension* caused by favouring a joint and protecting it from painful movements
- *stress* which can cause fatigue and depression, both of which can lead to increased levels of pain.

These factors form a vicious circle—inflammation and joint damage cause pain, which leads to muscle tension, stress, and increased pain. Unfortunately, diseases such as arthritis can wedge the 'pain gate' (a point in the spinal cord through which pain signals travel to the brain) open so that the sufferer experiences persistent, i.e. chronic, pain.

Stress and dwelling on pain, as well as the illness itself, is known to keep this pathway open. However, there are ways to close it. The body can produce its own pain killers, called endorphins (morphine-like substances), which shut the pain gate naturally. Release of these natural pain killers can be triggered by massage, heat and cold therapy, physiotherapy and exercise, as well as by medication. The pain gate can also be closed by using simple methods such as adopting a positive attitude to life, relaxation and distraction techniques, and meditation.

MEDICATIONS

Analgesics such as paracetamol or codeine often provide effective pain relief in osteoarthritis where there is no inflammation present. However, if joints are inflamed, either in osteo- or rheumatoid arthritis, then non-steroidal anti-inflammatory drugs may be prescribed. These can be highly effective, not only in relieving pain but in reducing the swelling and stiffness in the joint and increasing its mobility. It's important that these drugs are taken in strict accordance with the prescription because they can have adverse effects on the digestive system.

Many people, however, are reluctant to rely on chemical solutions over the long term and want non-pharmaceutical options for controlling their pain.

PHYSIOTHERAPY

One option for natural pain control is physical therapy. A physiotherapist can employ a number of techniques to reduce pain for arthritis sufferers, including ultrasound and electrical stimulation such as TENS (transcutaneous electric nerve stimulation) and diathermy, which are used in addition to a program of massage, joint mobilisation and posture correction.

Ultrasound is a technique which uses high-frequency sound waves to penetrate deep into tissue to reduce inflammation and ease pain. A conducting gel is spread over the affected area and the ultrasound wand is then gently moved back and forward over it. If the joint is bony such as in the hand or foot, then a water bath is used.

A TENS machine may sound like a weapon from *Star Wars* but is, in fact, a clever electronic device used to relieve pain. It works by stimulating various nerve pathways to the brain, which then encourages the body to release endorphins. It is commonly used by physiotherapists, but there are small portable models available from pharmacists for home use. If you are interested in buying one, discuss it with your physiotherapist first.

Diathermy uses microwaves or high-frequency electric currents to heat affected joints deep into the tissue, bringing rapid relief. The treatment is quite painless but is not suitable for all patients.

Laser light is also used by physiotherapists to relieve pain, reduce inflammation and promote healing. It is particularly helpful for tendons and small joints.

HEAT AND COLD THERAPY

Both heat and cold will close the pain gate, bringing quick relief to arthritis sufferers. This can be carried out by your physiotherapist, or by yourself at home. Home heat treatments include warm baths and showers, hot packs or water bottles and electric blankets. All simple to do, they can nevertheless bring comforting relief from nagging pain. Just make sure that whatever you use is not too hot—you want penetrating warmth, not burnt skin! Cold can be just as effective as heat and is especially good when inflammation is present. Ice cubes in a plastic bag, wrapped in a towel can be applied to the area but you can also buy special packs that can be kept in your freezer, handy for when you need them.

MASSAGE

Massage is an ancient and most relaxing therapy which eases muscle tension, reduces pain and promotes a sense of well-being. So if your budget permits, treat yourself to a session with a therapist qualified in remedial massage. Before they begin the therapist will ask you about your medical condition and assess the appropriate massage techniques to be used. The massage takes place in a warm, comfortable atmosphere and lasts for about an hour. Most people find that it has both physical and mental benefits.

You can also learn self-massage techniques such as gentle kneading or stroking of a painful muscle or joint. This is especially good for stiff necks, tight shoulder muscles, sore hands, elbows or knees. You can do it sitting in a chair or while you are having a warm bath. There are heat rubs and menthol gels which can aid self-massage so ask your pharmacist about the different types available. Do read the instructions carefully, though, because some are not designed to be followed by heat treatments. Always wash them off your skin after the massage.

EXERCISE AND PAIN MANAGEMENT

Exercise is a crucial part of any pain management program. Not only does it have health benefits like increasing fitness, promoting sleep and reducing stress but it also stretches the joint structures to relieve stiffness and pain, and restore flexibility. It also acts as a distraction—while you are exercising you are not focusing on your pain. Hydrotherapy is particularly good—your body feels light in the water and is able to move more freely than on dry land—and the warm water is comforting and promotes relaxation which has positive mental benefits.

STRESS AND PAIN PERCEPTION

Pain leads to stress, stress leads to depression, depression leads to an increased perception of pain. Symptoms of stress include:

- agitation
- short-temperedness
- loss of appetite
- sleeplessness
- tension
- anxiety.

These accumulated problems can be self-perpetuating, create a negative attitude and make your situation seem far blacker than it is. However, you can break this cycle. By learning to recognise when you are stressed then employing techniques to relieve it, you can reverse the pain/depression spiral, build a more positive outlook and reduce your pain perception.

A POSITIVE ATTITUDE TO LIFE

Scientific studies have proved that a positive outlook on life has both mental and physical benefits. It has been shown, for instance, that laughter boosts the immune system and promotes a sense of well-being and happiness. You may feel that there is nothing to laugh about in your situation, but there are ways to put humour in your path so that you are forced to trip over it.

According to Dr Patch Adams, who set up the Gesundheit Institute in America, medicine should be based on a loving, creative and above all humorous exchange. In his book, *Gesundheit!* (published by Healing Arts Press, Rochester, Vermont), he says, 'Research has shown that laughter increases the secretions of the natural chemicals, catecholamines and endorphins, that make people feel so peppy and good . . . Muscle physiologists have shown that anxiety and muscle relaxation cannot occur at the same time and that the relaxation response after a hearty laugh can last up to forty-five minutes.'

So even if you don't feel like laughing, put on a funny video, watch a comedy show or pick up a humorous book—it will do you the power of good.

RELAXATION

It is vital to learn effective relaxation techniques as they are a strong tool in the fight against pain. These techniques not only include generally relaxing activities such as social contact, going to the movies or even an evening stroll, but also specific things you can do to deal with acute pain and include:

- simple deep-breathing
- quieting the mind
- letting go of the body, muscle by muscle
- using visualisation.

In visualisation, you let your mind take you to a place of peace. This can be a real place where you have been happy, or some imaginary tranquil place. By visualising the serenity of the scene, your body will relax, your blood pressure will drop, tension will be released from your muscles and you'll experience a feeling of tranquillity. Your perception of pain will decrease and you'll feel in control and comfortable.

These techniques can be learned and, if practised daily, your quality of life will improve dramatically. Look in your community newspaper or ask the Arthritis Foundation in your state for information about relaxation classes near you.

MEDITATION

Meditation has been used through the ages to improve health and promote a feeling of well-being. Many people with acute illness and life threatening diseases have been helped by the power of meditation. There are various forms and it is really best to attend a class so that you can get direct instruction from a qualified teacher. You can then follow up at home with the use of books and meditation tapes.

DISTRACTION

This is the old-fashioned idea of 'taking your mind off it', but it can be extremely effective. If you dwell on your pain, the focused attention is going to intensify your perception of it. If you refocus your mind away from the pain onto something you enjoy, such as painting or creative writing, then your mind forgets about the pain and so your perception of it decreases.

PAIN MANAGEMENT PLAN

It is really important that you work out a pain management plan with the help of your doctors, physiotherapist, family and friends. Find out as much as possible about the various options of pain management, try different techniques and find out which ones work for you.

If you find it difficult to stay on top of your pain, then there are pain clinics in most major hospitals with specialists, counsellors and educators who are expert in this field. Ask your doctor for a referral. Also ask the Arthritis Foundation in your state about its 'self-management programs'. Whichever path you choose, make a commitment to:

- give any program you try a fair go
- not allow pain to rule your life
- accept pain as a challenge to be overcome.

Take heart—with all the medicines, treatments and techniques available today, pain can be controlled and quality of life maintained.

4

Relaxation and stress control

The word 'stress' entered popular vocabulary in the mid 1980s when it became almost fashionable to be 'stressed'—the word was like a badge for hard work. In fact, if you didn't claim to be stressed it was almost an admission of laziness.

Stress is a natural part of our lives. If we didn't experience stress—the 'fight or flight' response—we would never survive because we wouldn't react to danger, accidents or unsafe situations. When we are faced with stressful situations our bodies respond by increasing production of hormones such as adrenaline and cortisol which change our heart rate, blood pressure and metabolism, putting all systems on alert so we have the stamina to stand and fight or run away from any perceived danger. This was fine in the days when we faced sabre-toothed tigers or marauding vandals, because the effort involved in fighting or fleeing allowed the body to use up these substances and the reaction to subside when we were finally safe. We still have this survival response which can be triggered by real or perceived threats to safety, conflict, or unfamiliar circumstances such as:

- family, neighbour or work confrontations
- traffic problems

- feeling unsafe (on public transport, on lonely streets etc.)
- moving to an unfamiliar suburb
- changing jobs
- marriage
- birth of a child
- divorce
- death of a loved one (including the loss of a pet).

However, without the effort actually involved in a fight or taking flight, we have no natural mechanism to switch off this response automatically and over a period of time this 'stress' can lead to anxiety, depression, digestive problems, insomnia, loss of appetite and fatigue.

We all cope with stress in different ways. Some people thrive on being busy, love being at the centre of things, enjoy pressure, tight deadlines and sometimes even conflict. Other people prefer a more peaceful, orderly life and don't like conflict in any form.

Illness can also cause stress. If you are living with a chronic disease such as arthritis, which produces pain, stiffness in your joints, fatigue, depression and perhaps dependency on others, your whole system is permanently under stress, even though you might not be conscious of it.

There's a great deal we can do to manage stress, but firstly it's important to:

- recognise when you're stressed
- identify what causes you to be stressed
- learn how to reduce stress levels
- learn how to overcome the negative effects of stress
- learn how to relax
- learn peace of mind.

WHAT CAUSES YOU STRESS?

First of all, it's important to recognise when you are stressed. In stressful situations you may experience:

- an increase in your pulse rate
- a pounding heart

- faster breathing
- sweaty palms
- a clenched jaw.

Now think about all the times you experience these sensations. When do they happen? Make a list of the occasions when you think you are stressed—driving in heavy traffic, arguing with your children, dealing with bureaucracy, commuting, working with a difficult boss or colleague, watching the nightly TV news. Study the list and see which ones you can do something about. For instance, if traffic snarls and aggressive drivers intimidate you, think about taking an advanced driving course which will teach you how to handle a car more confidently and give you the skills to avoid dangerous situations on the road—or switch to public transport. If you have a teenage son or daughter with whom you are constantly fighting, then you could consult a family counsellor about ways to open up better communications between the two of you. If the nightly news leaves you feeling that the world is doomed—stop watching it. The point here is to look for solutions to the problem and then act on them. This will give you a feeling of being on top of the situation.

Keep a notepad and pen handy and write down every time you feel stressed, what happens, what caused it and how you feel about it. Adopt and practise the techniques suggested in this chapter and then use them to cope with the situation and note how you respond. You will soon be able to recognise the causes of your stress and develop appropriate techniques to deal with it.

LEARN TO RELAX

Relaxation—relieving muscular and mental tension—is one of the most powerful tools in overcoming the harmful effects of stress. Total relaxation is a technique which has to be learned and practised, but there are many classes available for you to join. Look in your local community newspaper, contact your local hospital, or enquire through the Arthritis Foundation about classes in your area.

Yoga, Tai Chi, visualisation and meditation are also good ways to relax the mind and body. There are many classes, tapes and videos available to help you learn these techniques, but it is sometimes easier to learn from a teacher who can answer any of your questions.

BETTER COMMUNICATION

Talking to someone you trust is one of the best ways to relieve tension and reduce stress. The old sayings 'a trouble shared is a trouble halved' and 'getting it all off your chest' have a lot of truth in them. Try talking to the person closest to you and listening to what they say. It may help put things into perspective. They may come up with good solutions to your problems, but simply sharing your concerns with another person can lighten the burden. If expressing yourself, discussing your feelings or opening up to another person is difficult for you, there are counsellors, courses and books on effective self-expression which may be able to help you.

If you have problems at work, try talking to the human resources officer or a colleague that you trust. If the problems are personal and you feel unable to confide in your family, then you could approach your doctor, clergyman or a family therapist for help.

KNOW YOUR LIMITATIONS

It's important not to have impossible expectations of yourself. It's all very well striving to be the best partner, father, mother, child, employee on the planet, but if that leaves you worn out and exhausted, you'll actually achieve less than if you'd simply 'done your best'. No-one expects you to be super human, so don't waste your precious energy trying to achieve the impossible. It's better to say 'no' to people, than agree to do something and end up feeling stressed, exhausted and maybe resentful. Respect your energy and stamina levels and don't push yourself beyond them. Come to terms with your capacities, ask for help when you need it—that way you'll not only look after yourself but your relationships too.

LEARN TO EXPRESS YOUR NEGATIVE FEELINGS WITHOUT HURTING OTHERS

The secret here is to say how you *feel* about something, rather than *accusing* someone of what you perceive as their shortcomings. For example, it's better to say, 'Cleaning the house makes me so tired and I feel hurt that it's always left to me', rather than, 'You'd never dream of lifting a finger around the house. You just expect me to act as your slave.'

When people angrily accuse someone they often make pointing gestures at the person with their index finger. In body language, this is like stabbing the other person, which automatically makes them defensive and they usually respond by hurling back an accusation of their own. The verbal duel that follows doesn't resolve anything.

If you tell someone how you *feel* about something, it invites them to express how they feel about it too, and they might respond to the situation with, 'I'm sorry, I thought you preferred to clean the house because I don't do it properly,' rather than 'What do you mean? I do just as much as you!' which leads to further argument. Learning to express yourself in this way will benefit all your relationships.

If you get really angry about something, give yourself time to cool down before tackling the person concerned. Go for a swim, listen to some music, watch a comedy video (it's very hard to maintain your rage while laughing), or do some gardening—anything you find soothing, that will give you time to think and examine both sides of the argument. Then, when you're calm and in control, you can talk about the situation rationally and deal with it.

OVERCOMING THE BLUES

Our outlook on life plays an influential role in the way we feel mentally, physically, and emotionally. When confident and happy, our stress levels will be low; when negative and miserable, our stress levels will rise. In the same way, how we perceive any illness will affect its outcome. If you believe that arthritis is something you are a 'martyr' to, then it's likely to have a much more debilitating effect than if you treat it as one of life's challenges which can be overcome.

The power of positive thinking can't be underestimated. If you focus on all the good things in your life you will feel happier, have more drive, be more enjoyable company and gain greater satisfaction from life. Allowing yourself to be overcome with self-pity will curb your motivation, elevate your sense of pain, increase fatigue and lead to a downward spiral of depression.

Depression is a recognised symptom of arthritis and one that it's important to overcome. Pain, decreased mobility, fears for the future, grief at no longer being able to participate in favoured activities, anger at the sense of having aged beyond your years are all common and understandable responses to this disease, but it's vital that you recognise and deal with these negative emotions.

Some people with arthritis will have clinical depression which needs proper treatment. The best approach when feeling despondent is to take responsibility for yourself, treat arthritis as a challenge, and see what you can do to beat it. Think about all the dreadful things which are *not* happening in your life (like war, starvation or plague), then focus on all the good things (like your loved ones, good food, music, art). Actively seek out pleasure in day-to-day things—there is a great deal of beauty and wonder all around us if we only care to see it (birds, flowers, children, animals). This may seem a bit Pollyanna-ish but it works!

If you find yourself slipping into despondency try expressing your feelings in song writing or poetry—it doesn't matter if it doesn't rhyme properly—as it's a great way to release pent-up emotions.

Take positive steps to improve your mood. If you're a woman, pamper yourself by having a massage, facial or new hair do. If you're a man, spend some time in your 'shed', go for a beer with a mate, pursue a favourite hobby. Treat yourself to some good food, visit a friend who makes you

laugh, or buy yourself a present—anything you find pleasurable.

Be as active as you can be. Visit family and friends; go
to the library, to the movies, the theatre; read widely; take
up something new like painting, a language, or a craft of
some kind—anything that will give you a new interest in
life and help you forget about your health and get on with
living.

Put some fun into your life

Laughter is a powerful medicine. Dr Patch Adams, the
celebrated American physician, says, 'Good health is a
laughing matter'. Dr Adams calls himself a social revolution-
ary who dispenses health care free of charge and with large
doses of humour at the Gesundheit Institute in West Virginia,
USA. As he says in the introduction to his book, *Gesundheit!*:

> . . . health is based on happiness—from hugging and
> clowning around to finding joy in family and friends,
> satisfaction in work, and ecstasy in nature and the
> arts—healing is not only prescribing medicine and ther-
> apies but working together and sharing in a spirit of joy.

Accept what you can't change

Your family and friends may not act or be exactly how you
would like, but they're not going to change no matter how
much you pressure or nag them. Accepting your partner,
parents or children for who they are will probably reduce
any tension between you and may improve your relationship.
Instead of becoming frustrated, tense and angry because they
haven't done what you wanted them to, try to smile, shrug
your shoulders and love them anyway.

Life isn't always fair

You only have to look around the world to see that life isn't
fair at times, so try not to let yourself slip into self-pity. Yes,
it's tough that you have arthritis and your siblings don't, and
your partner and children may not understand all that you

are going through, but these are the cards you've been dealt and maybe you don't understand the difficulties others are facing in their lives. Try to take life as it comes and make the best of it. This approach will not only have positive health benefits for you but will give you a sense of achievement when you reach the goals you set yourself.

A SIMPLE RELAXATION EXERCISE

Set aside 15–20 minutes each day for this relaxation exercise. Make sure you won't be interrupted and that there are no distractions.

1. Sit in a comfortable chair or lie down. Close your eyes and focus your mind on your toes. Flex them backwards and forwards, allowing the tension to ease each time you change directions. Then do the same with your whole foot. Slowly tense and relax all the muscles in your body working your way up from your toes to your face.
2. Next, breathe in and out slowly and rhythmically, saying to yourself, 'peace, serenity, tranquillity', slowly over and over again.
3. Once you feel comfortable and relaxed let your mind take you to a real or imagined place, somewhere beautiful where you feel comfortable and safe. In your mind, look around at the beautiful scenery—perhaps waves gently lapping on white sand, sunlight dancing on a crystal clear creek, butterflies dancing through a rain forest.
4. Your relaxation period should last for about 15–20 minutes. Ask someone to gently rouse you after that time, or set a clock radio to come on quietly, tuned to a soft music station. Whatever you choose it should be gentle, not abrupt like an alarm. Many people find that their internal clock tells them when the time is up and they rouse just before they are called.

Try to practise every day. If you do you'll find it easier and easier to relax your mind and body. Many people find that after a while they can relax at will, anywhere, any time.

Relaxation will help you gain better control of your arthritis, help you overcome pain, feel more positive about life and bring greater happiness into it. So try to:

- set aside some relaxing time each day
- find a method which suits you
- release muscle tension throughout the day by tensing and relaxing muscles in your neck, face, shoulders, hands and legs.

If you find yourself feeling tense during the day take a break, close your eyes, breathe slowly and evenly, and let your mind take you to your special place—even for just a few minutes.

USE SUPPORT SERVICES

There are many organisations and institutions, such as the Arthritis Foundation, local hospitals, community groups and adult education centres, which run courses and workshops that can help you learn to deal with stress. In joining one of these programs you will meet other people in a similar situation and talking about your shared experiences can help you cope with your own problems in a positive way.

5

Beating fatigue

Next to pain, fatigue is the second biggest problem that arthritis sufferers have to deal with. Like pain, the perception of fatigue varies from person to person—from a mild lack of energy to the sensation of complete exhaustion, where muscles feel weak, every action seems an effort, you have difficulty performing the simplest tasks, and even lying in bed seems tiring. Fatigue is especially common in the autoimmune forms such as rheumatoid arthritis and SLE (lupus). Feelings of fatigue include:

- total lack of energy
- compulsion to lie down
- listlessness
- drowsiness
- lack of motivation
- lethargy
- simple tasks becoming a major effort.

When tired, our perception of pain increases, and coping with pain can increase our fatigue. Pain and fatigue can lead to depression which in turn increases the pain and tiredness. This may make you feel:

- helpless
- out of control
- unable to concentrate on anything
- unable to make decisions

- irritable
- uncooperative.

Overcoming fatigue is an important step in managing any form of arthritis and, fortunately, there are strategies you can use to beat it and put energy back into your life.

WHY AM I SO TIRED?

With arthritis, fatigue is caused by physical, emotional and environmental factors, which include:

- *pain*—three aspects of pain can cause fatigue. Coping with the pain itself can be physically and mentally draining, leaving you tired and listless. Also, if your joints are painful you may be holding them in a position of least pain, causing the surrounding muscles to spasm and become fatigued. Lastly, pain may be preventing you from sleeping well, which leads to exhaustion the next day.
- *lack of exercise*—there is a close relationship between fatigue and exercise. If you exercise you'll have more energy; the less active you become, the more tired you'll feel. If your body lacks regular exercise your muscles become weaker so that simple everyday living is tiring. It's one of the reasons why exercise is so important in dealing with arthritis. Of course, if you over-exercise at any one time you're going to feel tired at the end of it, but this short-term fatigue is not the same as the long-term exhaustion caused by arthritis and inactivity.
- *depression*—it's well recognised that living with a chronic illness can cause depression through coping with pain, difficulty moving around and performing everyday chores, and not having the lifestyle you once had. Depression robs you of motivation—it just seems too much bother to do anything or go anywhere. As a result you become lethargic, which makes you even less motivated to do anything. This in turn contributes to your depression and sense of fatigue. You may develop a negative outlook on life, and negative emotions will drain you of energy.

- *stress*—a number of environmental factors can cause stress which results in fatigue. If joints are painful, simple day-to-day tasks such as waiting in a bank queue or at the supermarket checkout can be stressful, leading to agitation, bad temper and fatigue. Climbing stairs, housework, cooking, any number of everyday events can prove stressful when you are in pain or can't manage physically as well as you used to. One symptom of this kind of stress is exhaustion.
- *noise*—exposure to unpleasant, constant or loud noise can be extremely wearing if you're coping with a chronic illness, especially if you're unable to do anything about it. Traffic noise, a barking dog, loud rock music, a persistent car alarm going off (especially if it makes a high pitched screeching noise), can be intolerable to many people suffering from arthritis and if exposed to it over a period of time can leave them feeling wrung out.
- *the weather*—either too hot and humid or too cold. Many people find their joints become swollen and painful when certain weather conditions prevail. For some people it's cold weather which triggers a flare-up, leaving them exhausted; for others it's hot humid weather which robs them of energy.
- *flare-ups*—whenever arthritis is in an active phase then fatigue is usually one of the first symptoms.

WHAT CAN I DO ABOUT IT?

As everyone experiences fatigue at different times and from different causes, it is important for you to work out what it is that makes you tired. Keep a record for at least two weeks, on the chart on pages 44–5, of the times you feel tired and what you think was the cause. Once you have kept this chart for two weeks, see if there is a pattern to your tiredness. Itemise the things you think have contributed to your fatigue and see if you can do something about them. For example, do you feel tired every morning on waking? If so, you may not be getting enough quality sleep and may have to adopt strategies to improve your night's rest. Maybe

Fatigue chart

Day	Depression	Flare-ups	Noise	Pain	Stress	Weather	Other
Monday							
times							
Tuesday							
times							
Wednesday							
times							
Thursday							
times							
Friday							
times							
Saturday							
times							
Sunday							
times							

Day	Depression	Flare-ups	Noise	Pain	Stress	Weather	Other
Monday							
times							
Tuesday							
times							
Wednesday							
times							
Thursday							
times							
Friday							
times							
Saturday							
times							
Sunday							
times							

you feel tired after having visitors; if so, it may be a good idea to cut back the visits or arrange them for a time when you're feeling most energetic.

STRATEGIES TO GIVE YOURSELF MORE ENERGY

- Improve your posture and movements. Talk to your physiotherapist about the best ways to stand, sit or move around for your condition, so that you put the least stress on painful joints.
- Work at keeping a good balance between activity and rest. Respect your body's signals—when you feel tired it's important to rest. Pushing on regardless is just going to make you more exhausted.
- Organise your day so that work and rest periods are alternated. Do work you find most tiring at times when you have most energy.
- Slow down when a flare-up strikes; do only what you have to and rest frequently.
- Respect your energy levels. Never give yourself tight deadlines to complete work or projects. It will only put pressure on you to continue working past the point where you need to rest. Pushing on will cause increased strain on your joints and make you feel exhausted.
- Plan ahead and organise your time efficiently. Eliminate any work that isn't absolutely necessary. Delegate tasks both at home and at work—this isn't a sign of weakness, it's actually good management practice. Each night, make a list of all the things you have to do next day, then prioritise them. Work out which ones might be tiring, then alternate them with less tiring ones, and remember to include regular rest periods throughout the day.
- Use labour saving devices at work and at home such as word processors, electric can openers, automatic garage doors, etc.
- Buy utensils and tools with padded grips and long handles. The Independent Living Centre in your state capital can provide you with information on manufacturers or distributors of this type of equipment.

GETTING A GOOD NIGHT'S SLEEP

The most important factor in getting a good night's sleep is to have a firm yet comfortable bed—one which gives you good support, yet feels relaxing to be in. Many arthritis patients find lamb's wool or sheepskin underlays very soothing. Sleep with only one pillow which supports your head but keeps your neck horizontal. Make sure that you don't have doonas or heavy blankets which make you too warm during the night. Being too warm in bed can prevent you going into deep sleep, which is the most restorative kind. Here are nine ways to get a better night's sleep.

- Try to go to bed at the same time every night and get up at the same time every morning. This accustoms your body to sleeping and waking in a natural pattern.
- Develop a routine in going to bed. If you follow the same ritual of activities—like washing your face, brushing your hair, cleaning your teeth—it signals to your mind that you're preparing for sleep; this can improve your ability to drift off to sleep quickly and easily.
- It's best not to use alcohol as a sedative and avoid tea, coffee or any other caffeinated drinks in the evening. Smoking less than an hour and a half before retiring can make it harder to fall asleep.
- Try to make yourself as comfortable as possible in bed. If you are in pain, then take some analgesic. Don't rely on sleeping pills for a good night's sleep—while they can be helpful in the short term, they don't promote quality sleep and can contribute to some people's sleeping problems.
- Bed is not a good place to deal with your worries. Discipline yourself to think about problems, or any concerns you have, for a set time during the day; make decisions on how you can resolve them, take steps to do this and then put them out of your mind.
- If you're unable to fall asleep, get up again and read a book or listen to some music. Go back to bed only when you're feeling sleepy.
- Try to reduce noise levels in your bedroom by closing

windows, curtains and doors; wearing ear-plugs can also help.

- Try to get enough exercise during the day. Regular exercise improves the quality of sleep.
- If you feel tired, don't be too proud to ask for help. Your partner, family and friends will much prefer to have you up and about than flat on your back in bed because you've taken on too much.

Fatigue isn't something you have to put up with—there's plenty you can do about it. If you are feeling more tired than normal, talk to your doctor as it could be a sign that your arthritis is active. Remember, you can fight fatigue better if you pace yourself, tune in to what your body is telling you, rest when you're tired, exercise when you're well, ask for help and follow your management plan. If you do all this you may find you have more energy than you've had in years!

6

Keeping your sex life alive

When the subject of arthritis is discussed, sex is rarely part of the topic. Somehow it's not considered appropriate. But we are all sexual creatures and whether we have a health problem or not, we still have sexual needs and desires. Because arthritis affects the joints, you may find that favoured positions for lovemaking become difficult or painful. If you live with pain, you may not feel as sexually responsive to your partner as they would like you to be. Arthritis may also leave you *feeling* less attractive than you were which can also impact on your relationship.

No matter what type of arthritis you have it will be affecting one or more joints, most likely the knees, hips, back, shoulder or finger joints. Trouble in the bedroom can lead to marital problems when there is no disease present, let alone when you are living with a chronic illness! Painful, stiff joints are not conducive to relaxed or animated lovemaking, but both you and your partner may still crave the sensuality, intimacy and gratification that comes from sex. Sex is a subject which should be talked about in the context of arthritis so you can deal with any difficulties which might arise and find ways of overcoming them.

SEXUAL PROBLEMS

Sexual problems fall into three main areas—lack of sexual desire, finding a comfortable position and lack of communication between partners. Be aware of the following problems:

- pain, stiffness or poor body-image can lower libido in many arthritis sufferers, especially women
- even if there is a strong sexual desire, joint pain from certain positions can either kill or interfere with the pleasure of lovemaking
- lack of communication between partners can lead to misunderstanding
- your partner may feel inhibited because they don't want to hurt you
- your partner may be doing something that is causing you pain, but you feel you can't tell them to stop.

These elements can all lead to tension in the relationship, which impacts on your sex life, which adds to the tensions—it's a vicious circle.

LACK OF SEXUAL DESIRE

Putting aside sadomasochism, pain is a sure-fire killer of sexual desire for most people. It's difficult to become sexually aroused when you are experiencing pain because your mind will be preoccupied with the pain rather than sexual excitement. The brain is the most important sex organ we have. What's going on in your mind has far more impact on whether you get sexually aroused than any physical stimulation. Even if you're enjoying sex play, but have at the back of your mind the idea that maybe you'll be required to get into a position or do something which could hurt, then it's going to hold you back.

If you've experienced pain during intercourse in the past, you may be reluctant to make love to your partner in case it happens again. If you feel guilty about this and don't discuss it with your partner, you'll set up mental and emotional barriers between you, which may be hard to break down. Many people in this situation withdraw from all intimate contact with their partner in case it sends the wrong signals. As a result, their partner feels bewildered, rejected, confused and unhappy, which just compounds the problem. We all need physical closeness and intimacy—touching, stroking, kissing and cuddling are comforting and reassuring gestures. We know how much babies and children need this intimate physical contact and suppose, wrongly, that we grow out of it. It's true that most of us don't need the same degree of physical reassurance as a child, but we do need physical affection, especially when we're dealing with a chronic illness.

Communication is vitally important here. Try talking to your partner about the way you feel, what you're experiencing during sex, and then *listen* to what they have to say. (If you find talking about sex with your partner difficult, then you could approach the Family Planning Association which offers counselling on sexual matters as well as contraception.) Maybe you can try different positions and experiment to find which are most comfortable. Maybe you need some extra stimulation, such as a vibrator, to heighten your arousal. There are a whole host of things you could try. And simply dealing with the problem together, rather than shutting your partner out, can create a stronger sense of intimacy which will be beneficial in itself.

SELF-ESTEEM

Arthritis can cause physical changes in the body which may affect the way you look and move. You may feel you've aged beyond your years because you're no longer as flexible and nimble as you once were. Pain, fatigue and stress may be showing in your face and posture, so that when you look at yourself in the mirror you don't see yourself as attractive any more.

There's a funny aspect to human sexuality: if we feel attractive, there's a certain 'something' about us that *is* attractive. Look what happens when we fall in love—it has a physical effect on us. Our eyes shine, our skin glows, we have a lightness to our step. If you allow arthritis to 'get you down', then it will also show in your physical appearance. If you believe you are no longer sexually attractive, you may become less attractive.

Society also contributes to the problem. Community attitudes seem to follow the advertising notion that 'sex is only for young, able-bodied and beautiful people'. This not only causes a great deal of pain and misery to young people who don't conform to the slim, smooth-muscled, beautiful image of sexual attractiveness, but to most people with health problems such as arthritis. Our society seems to be telling us that sex is not for the fat, ugly, disabled, sick or old. It denies the fact that we are all sexual creatures and should be able to express ourselves sexually without being made to feel ashamed or embarrassed about it. If we are having problems with sex then we should be able to seek help to overcome them. Many people with arthritis don't like to admit to their partners that they are experiencing difficulty with sex, let alone to their doctors. This lack of communication can compound the situation in several ways.

For the man

If a man has arthritis, pain may prevent him gaining or keeping an erection, which in turn may make him anxious about becoming impotent. If you have not been able to get or sustain an erection for some time, the best thing you can do is just forget about it. Don't set yourself the goal of having intercourse in your sex life. Realise that you can bring your partner to climax, if that's what she wants, without having to have an erection at all. You can use your hands and mouth and for lots of women this is actually more pleasurable than intercourse. If you stop concentrating on having an erection, it will probably 'turn up'.

If you are suffering from performance anxiety (whether you can be a good lover to your partner), then you should just relax and have some fun without turning lovemaking into an event where you'll be judged. Talk to your partner about the pressure you feel under to 'perform'. Explain that you'd like to simply 'fool around' and just want to pleasure her and have her pleasure you.

If your problems persist, don't just suffer in silence. Men's general and sexual health is much more openly discussed these days and there are many ways you can seek help. Talk to your family doctor, who can refer you to a urologist to see if there is any physical cause for your problems. If you want greater anonymity you could contact one of the many new men's health centres which specialise in helping men overcome sexual problems. The Family Planning Association also offers sexual counselling for singles and couples, so perhaps both you and your partner can talk to one of their therapists.

For the woman

Women can feel particularly anxious about physical changes to their appearance, to the point where they don't like to be seen naked anymore. Maybe they've put on weight because they are no longer as active as they once were. Maybe when they look in the mirror they just see a pale drawn face rather than the attractive, vital woman they used to see. Maybe they just feel too tired for sex. All this can build into a poor self-image which can have a major impact on a couple's sex life.

Many men say that even though they still find their partners extremely attractive, the woman can't be convinced because she's measuring herself against the artificial notion, as portrayed in the media, of what makes a woman beautiful. Again it's important that both partners talk openly and honestly about the way they feel. It's especially important for a woman to *listen* to her man, rather than presupposing that he too believes the media myth of what a beautiful woman is.

Don't lose sight of yourself

Accepting that you have arthritis and that there are ways to overcome any problems that arise, will go a long way toward making you feel back in control. There are ways to keep you as flexible as possible (in fact, some people with arthritis who follow a recommended exercise program end up much more flexible than they were before they were diagnosed with the disease). Keeping yourself well-groomed will also boost your self-esteem. Buying new clothes, treating yourself to a facial, massage or whatever form of pampering you enjoy will also help to make you feel better about yourself and this will be reflected in your looks and attitude.

BETTER COMMUNICATION

Sharing your feelings and concerns with your partner and listening to theirs can lead to a greater sense of intimacy between you. If you understand one another, you can work on ways to improve sex for both of you. Maybe new positions would overcome the problem, maybe you need more spontaneity or romance in your life. If you've been together for a long time, you may have fallen into a regular pattern of lovemaking which is no longer inspiring under these new circumstances. Whatever the cause, the problem should be talked through and solutions found.

- Talk to your partner about your sex life—but wait until you're alone and won't be interrupted.
- Try something new—a different place and time, a sex toy or vibrator, rather than just going through the same old routine when you go to bed at night.
- Talk about one another's fantasies and maybe get a fantasy going between you.
- Explain what turns you on and encourage your partner to tell you what they like.
- Experiment with different positions to see what feels good. You never know, you may discover an exciting position you've never tried before.
- Agree on a prearranged code word to let your partner know if something is painful for you. Sometimes, at the height of excitement, moans and groans can be misinterpreted as sounds of ecstasy.

- Take turns in stroking and massaging one another.
- Tell your partner whenever they are doing something you particularly enjoy.
- Plan for sex—it doesn't always have to be spontaneous. You can aim for intercourse at a time when you know you'll be feeling your best. Time your analgesics so that they're working during your lovemaking. Have a warm bath or shower together to relax your muscles and heighten your feelings of sensuality.
- Discuss what you can and can't do with your doctors if you have had hip or knee replacement surgery.
- Stroking, fondling, kissing, sucking, can all be done without much effort—even if you can no longer take a 'vigorous' role in lovemaking it doesn't mean your partner has to do all the work.

Having to deal with changes in your lovemaking can have positive outcomes if it leads to better communication, the discovery of new and exciting positions and techniques, and a renewed sense of intimacy between you. So turn a negative into a positive and enjoy yourselves! There is a lot you can do to put the *zing* back into your sex life.

7

Taking the strain off your joints

When you have arthritis it's extremely important to take care of your joints. If stressed, inflamed swollen joints can be damaged more easily, leading to further degeneration of their structure. So it's vital for you to learn how to sit, stand, walk and handle things in a way that puts the least strain on your joints. It's not difficult, it just means doing things a little differently.

- When lifting or carrying heavy objects, distribute the weight over the strongest joints, and use large muscle groups, such as your thighs, instead of your back. For example, if you're lifting a heavy object, bend your knees, keep your back straight and use your thigh muscles to lift.
- When carrying shopping or heavy bags, place the handles over your forearm instead of your fingers, hands or wrists. In fact, it's a good idea to use a string bag for shopping which has a large strap so that you can carry it on your shoulder.
- If using your hands to push yourself up from a sitting to a standing position, use your palms to take the weight.
- When closing doors, drawers or cupboards, use your hip instead of your hands.

- If the height of your kitchen benches forces you to stoop while working at them, place a thick wooden chopping block on the bench to create a raised working area.

GRIPPING AND TURNING

Gripping and turning actions place considerable stress on the joints of your hands. Here are some suggestions to help:

- Use an electric can opener if possible.
- Use a jar top opener fixed to the underside of an overhead kitchen cupboard (there are several types available).
- Choose the lever variety of taps, which can be used with your forearm, if necessary, rather than the conventional type of tap if fitting out a new kitchen or bathroom.

SITTING

- Avoid staying in one position for too long. Get up every 20–30 minutes and stretch, walk around the room or do some range-of-motion exercises (see Chapter 9) for a few minutes.
- Sit in a chair with a firm, yet comfortable and supportive, back and seat. If it's a lounge chair, it should have arms so you can rest your arms on them. If it's a desk chair it should be armless so that you can draw it close to the desk.
- Sit in a chair with your bottom at the back of the seat, your lower back supported either by the chair, a back support roll or a rolled up towel.
- When sitting, your feet should be flat on the ground or supported by a small foot stool so that your knees are slightly higher than your hips.
- Every now and then do a body audit—that is, think about how you are holding your body. Is your jaw clenched? If so do a wide yawn and then relax your jaw. How about your shoulders? Are they hunched and tense? If so, raise them towards your ears, then let them gently

drop down and relax them. Do this several times if they are very tense. Flex and tense your hands, flex and tense your feet. Go down through your body and see if you are holding any part of it in a tense way and, if so, release it by stretching, tensing and relaxing it.

STANDING

- Try not to stand for any length of time. This may not always be possible, especially if your job entails being on your feet, however, there are ways to minimise the strain.
- Always stand with your feet slightly apart so that the weight of your body is distributed down both legs.
- Don't lock your knees but keep them slightly bent and relaxed.
- If possible place one foot on a raised object to reduce the strain on your legs and lower back, changing feet from time to time. If you're in the kitchen open a cupboard door and place your foot on the bottom shelf. If behind a counter, then an upturned empty box will do.

WALKING

Whether walking for exercise or simply to the shops or bus stop, remember to do the following:

- Keep your shoulders back and your head up.
- Swing your arms freely with your hands relaxed.
- Swing your stride from the hip, not the knee. It should be a relaxed, rhythmic movement, not a shuffle.
- Wear comfortable, well-supporting shoes.
- Give yourself enough time to walk at a comfortable pace for you. Scurrying on hard pavements can stress the joints in your feet, ankles, knees and hips.

HOUSEWORK

- Try to simplify tasks. When cleaning the house leave a box at the top of the stairs, or at one end of the house, and put everything in it that has to be taken downstairs, or to the other end of the house, instead of making several trips.

- Use a workman's or gardener's tool holder to carry all the cleaning and polishing products that you need and carry it from place to place on your forearm.
- Buy the lightest vacuum cleaner (that will still do the job) you can find. Pushing and pulling a heavy monster can not only place strain on your joints but can tire you out as well.
- Dust using the suction hose and bristle head on your vacuum cleaner. Not only it is more efficient in removing the dust, but it cuts down the amount of hand movements required to do the job.
- Instead of dusting china and glass ornaments, rinse them in warm water with a dash of detergent in it, then let them dry naturally—it's less work and gets the dust out of all those nooks and crannies.
- When replacing ovens and fridges, buy self-cleaning and automatic defrosting models.
- Use fitted sheets and doonas on beds—bed making is much easier that way.
- If you can't get someone else to clean the bath, try using a sponge mop and cream cleanser to do the job—it saves all that bending over and rubbing.

COOKING

- There are many kitchen utensils on the market today designed to take the strain off joints. They have specially moulded and padded handles to make the action of the implement more efficient and reduce the amount of pressure or strength required to use it. They are available in the kitchen department of quality variety and department stores and kitchen specialty shops, or ask the Independent Living Centre in your state for more information.
- Place all heavy equipment at middle level in your kitchen

so that you neither have to lift it down nor raise it up to use it.

- Use labour saving devices such as electric blenders, choppers, graters and mixers. Many of these functions can be found in single appliances these days.
- When cooking a meal that freezes well, make a double quantity—one to eat straight away and one for another day.
- Plan ahead and cook at the weekend for the week ahead—you may have more energy then and other family members can help.
- Frozen vegetables are just as healthy as fresh ones and take a lot less preparation.

GARDENING

There are now many tools on the market which can make gardening easier for people with arthritis. Ask at your local nursery, or contact the Independent Living Centre in your state.

- Try to avoid kneeling for too long as this puts considerable strain on your knees.
- Use 'no dig' gardening methods to simplify bed preparation.
- Create raised beds where possible so that you can sit to garden.
- If weeding, sit on a low stool with your knees apart and bend forward at the hips, keeping your back straight. This helps take the strain off your back and knees.
- Use long handled tools whenever possible.

SPLINTS

Another way to save your joints is to rest them when they are inflamed. Often the best way to do this is to wear a splint, not only when you're resting but working too. Many people resist wearing splints as they think they make them look disabled. However, splints do an effective job in helping to protect your joints from further damage, helping prevent deformities and speeding recovery from 'flare-ups'. The same is true of crutches or walking sticks, which help to reduce the weight carried by inflamed or weakened joints such as the knees. Younger people, especially, resist their use, feeling that it makes them look old. But you should forget about image and be practical—it's better to preserve your joint than worry about what others might think.

INDEPENDENT LIVING CENTRES

As the name suggests, these centres have been set up in all capital cities of Australia to help the disabled, the aged and people suffering from debilitating diseases such as arthritis, to maintain independent lives. They offer impartial advice on a comprehensive range of aids and equipment including:

- bathroom and toilet equipment
- kitchen designs
- household products
- clothing and footwear
- communication devices
- lifting equipment
- leisure and recreation equipment
- seating
- transport.

Each centre has a team of health professionals, including occupational therapists and physiotherapists, who can discuss your needs and everyday problems. The centres also have mobile units which offer a travelling information service to country areas.

WHERE TO GO FOR MORE HELP

It's a good idea to talk to an occupational therapist for more specific information and advice on your personal needs for aids and special equipment. You could ask your doctor to refer you to an occupational therapist in your area.

Your physiotherapist can also give you information about

performing specific tasks or functions you might be having difficulty with and some local hospitals run classes on the subject. The Arthritis Foundation has brochures and information which could help and, as mentioned above, the Independent Living Centres have been set up for this specific purpose. (See page 175 for addresses and telephone numbers.)

8

How exercise can help you

Health experts tell us that exercise is a vital component of good health for everyone, but it's even more important for those suffering from arthritis, as it not only builds general health and fitness but also prevents joint stiffness, reduces swelling, and maintains strength and tone in the surrounding muscles, tendons and ligaments. It's the reason for the Arthritis Foundation's advice to 'Move it or lose it' if you want to relieve pain, prevent joint deformity, reduce stress, depression and dependence on others—quite a list of reasons for putting some activity into your day.

When people are diagnosed with arthritis their reaction is often to 'save' their joints in the belief that a deteriorating joint can be 'worn out' by exercise. However, becoming less active is the worst thing you can do and may exacerbate the problem. It's true that rest is required to soothe inflamed joints, but too much rest will lead to muscle weakness, increased stiffness and reduced mobility. There is a crucial balance to be learned between rest and exercise—when the joint is hot, inflamed and painful it should be rested, when it is not it should be exercised.

THE REST AND EXERCISE BALANCE

It's important to learn when to exercise, when to rest and how to move your joints in an appropriate way to minimise damage and maintain flexibility. You should:

- rest inflamed joints—which doesn't always mean bed rest; it can also mean doing a different activity, changing your posture, or wearing a splint
- exercise stiff joints—which can be done through gentle exercise such as swimming, walking, hydrotherapy or through mobilisation by your physiotherapist
- support weak or unstable joints—by wearing a splint, or using a walking stick or crutches
- relax—which will not only relieve muscle tension and stress but improve your mental outlook and make resting more effective.

Regular exercise will:

- reduce pain
- maintain or increase joint mobility
- relieve muscle tension
- improve sleep
- help with weight control
- improve your cardiovascular system
- strengthen bones and help prevent osteoporosis
- reduce stress levels
- improve your mental attitude
- enable you to look positively on life.

GUIDELINES FOR EXERCISE

There are two types of exercise you should build into your program. The first is general exercise to increase fitness such as walking, cycling, or swimming. The second is specific exercise to take your joints through their range of motion.

General exercise

- Set aside 20–30 minutes, 3–4 times each week.
- Use smooth, rhythmic movements rather than jerky ones.

- Respect pain and stop any exercise that hurts. (The only exception to this is gentle stretching where muscle pain may be felt.)
- If pain persists for more than two hours after exercising, you've done too much and should drop back a level on your program.
- Warm up before exercising by doing some simple stretching exercises, which not only prevents injury but increases the effectiveness of the exercise as muscles and joints are more responsive when warm.

A word of caution: if you've had a joint replaced, ask your surgeon or physiotherapist about which movements you can and can't do.

WHAT EXERCISE SHOULD I DO?

Walking

Walking is one of the best exercises for overall fitness and weight control because it gives your whole body a good aerobic workout. Walking uses almost all of the body's joints and muscles and is especially good for the major muscles of the upper and lower legs and buttocks. It will also strengthen back and abdominal muscles groups.

Try to achieve a pace where you can still comfortably hold a conversation. Keep your shoulders back and your head up. Swing your arms freely with your hands relaxed. As you gain stamina, increase your pace. You'll find the level at which you can just hold a conversation has increased in proportion to your fitness level.

Cycling

Cycling is a low impact exercise and good for developing cardiovascular fitness. It can be done on either a road or mountain bike or on a stationary bike if you don't feel confident enough to take to the open road. Cycling uses most of the major muscles in your legs but has limited benefit for the upper body.

When cycling, make sure you don't slouch. Keep your back straight with arms and shoulders relaxed. Don't lock your elbows, keep them relaxed and slightly bent. When pedalling, keep the pressure of the ball of your foot on the pedal a constant throughout the entire circle. It should be a circular motion, not a pumping one.

You should also use 'easy' gears as this will increase the aerobic benefit and reduce the chance of knee pain.

Most people new to cycling make the mistake of having the saddle too low, which can cause knee pain. If you have any doubts, check with the staff at your local bike shop.

Swimming, aquarobics, hydrotherapy

Swimming, aquarobics and hydrotherapy in warm water are good ways to exercise because the water takes the weight off your joints so they can move more easily. Exercise in water improves cardiovascular fitness and muscle tone. If swimming, try to use as many different strokes as you can as each stroke uses different muscle groups. Swimming will strengthen your arms, shoulders, chest, legs and buttocks. Aquarobics and hydrotherapy will also improve your muscle tone and strength by supporting your joints, muscles and body weight and allowing them to be taken through a greater range-of-motion, thus increasing mobility and flexibility.

Six water exercises to try

1. Walk the length of the pool, using your arms to pull you through the water in a breast-stroke fashion. Then walk backwards, scooping the water behind you to help make your passage easier.
2. Step sideways through the water, bringing your feet together with each step. Do 10 steps to the left, then 10 steps to the right.
3. Standing in shoulder-deep water, try marching through the water, lifting your knees as high as you can. Once you can do this easily, try running through the water.
4. Stand in shoulder-deep water and hold your arms straight out in front of you at shoulder height, with palms facing

out. Push your arms out and to the side, feeling the resistance of the water against your palms. Turn your palms in and bring your hands back together, keeping your arms at shoulder height. Repeat 5–10 times.

5. Treading water is also a good all-over workout, but especially good for the abdominals.
6. Stand with your back against the side of the pool with your arms lying along the pool edge. Lift your legs to hip height and bring them together, then push them apart. Repeat 4–5 times. This is especially good for the inner thighs.

EXERCISE COMBINATIONS

To maximise the benefits of exercise it's a good idea to do different exercises over the course of the week. This not only maintains your interest but makes sure that all your muscles and joints are given a full workout. A program that includes walking, swimming and cycling will provide a total body workout, improve cardiovascular fitness, improve muscle tone, and increase flexibility.

Remember, it's important to start slowly and build up gradually to maximise the benefits. If new to exercise, start with a 10-minute exercise period, adding five minutes to the time each week until you are exercising for at least 30 minutes. Once you have reached this goal use the following as a guide to combining your exercises.

Sunday	20–30 minute walk
Monday	30 minute stretching program
Tuesday	Rest
Wednesday	30 minute cycle
Thursday	40 minute aquarobics
Friday	Rest
Saturday	20–30 minute walk

Keeping an exercise chart is a good way of setting and reaching fitness goals while encouraging you to keep to your program. Aim for 3–4 times a week but not when your joints are inflamed or when you are feeling unwell. Keep a record on the following chart of what you complete each week. Mark W for walking, S for swimming, R for resting etc. and the time undertaken.

It's important to remember that when you first start to exercise you are making your body work harder than it's used to—your breathing will become heavier, your heart rate will increase and your muscles will be worked in a way they probably haven't been for years—so you may feel quite tired afterwards. However, you will probably wake next morning with renewed energy. As your program progresses your body will adapt to this amount of exercise, so that you will be able to increase the pace and duration of the exercise. Slowly but surely your muscles will tone up and strengthen, you'll become more flexible, your cardiovascular system will improve and your whole body will start to look and feel better.

If after exercise you feel pain for more than two hours, or you feel pain or over-tired the next day, then you have overdone it. Drop your program back to a level which you feel comfortable with for a few days and then increase it gradually again. Slow and steady increments are the secret of success.

SIMPLE DAILY STRETCHES

You can do these exercises in bed each morning before you get up.

1. Lie flat on your back, legs straight and arms by your side, feet pointing to the ceiling. Without moving your foot, curl your toes away from you, then pull them up towards you. Repeat 5–10 times.
2. Now point your feet down towards the end of the bed, then pull them up towards you. Repeat 5–10 times.
3. Next, keeping your leg straight and flat on the bed, pull your foot up, tightening your thigh muscles and stiffening your knee. Hold for a count of 5. Do each leg 2–5 times.
4. Still lying on your back, tighten your buttock muscles. Hold for a count of 5. Repeat 2–3 times.

Week	Monday	Tuesday	Wednesday	Thursday	Friday	Saturday	Sunday	Total
Target								
1								
2								
3								
4								
5								
6								
7								
8								
9								
10								

5. Now raise your knees up so that your feet are flat on the bed, with your hands by your sides. Push your lower back into the bed so that your pelvis tilts towards you. Hold for a count of 5. Repeat 5–10 times.

6. Relax your body and straighten your legs again. Now press your shoulders into the bed. Hold for a count of 5. Relax, then repeat 5 times.

7. Lie on your back with your knees bent, feet flat on the bed. Clasp your hands and lift your arms over your head as far as they will go. Gently bring them back to the starting position. Repeat 5 times.

8. Lie straight again with your hands by your sides, palms up, then bring your hands up to touch your shoulders. Lower them back down to the bed. Repeat 5–10 times.

9. Spread your legs as far as they will go. Turn your feet and legs out and then in. Repeat 5–10 times.

10. Lie on your back, draw your knees up so that your shins are horizontal and hold them with your hands for support behind your knees. Hold for a count of 10. Now keeping your legs in the same position, spread your arms out to the sides and gently rock your legs from side to side, keeping your shoulders flat to the bed.

11. Lying on your back, knees bent, feet flat to the bed, clasp under one knee with both hands and pull it towards your chest. Hold for a count of 10, then lower your leg to the bed and repeat with the other leg. Repeat 2–3 times each leg.

12. Sitting on the side of the bed, raise your left arm up and stretch up to the ceiling. Lower your arm and repeat with the right arm. Repeat 3–4 times each side.

13. Still sitting on the side of the bed, raise both arms and stretch to the ceiling, turn your palms out and slowly bring your arms down to your sides.

14. Sit on a chair with straight back and hands in your lap. Now, straighten your leg so that the muscles on the top of your thigh tighten. Lower your leg. Repeat 10 times, then change legs and repeat 10 times. Slowly build the number of leg raises until you can do 50 with each leg.

15. Sit on a chair with straight back and hands in your lap. Straighten your leg so that the muscles on the top of your thigh tighten. Keeping your leg in this position, point your toes, then pull them back towards you. Repeat 5 times. Now, circle your toes to the left 5 times, then to the right 5 times. Lower your foot to the ground and repeat with your other leg.

RANGE-OF-MOTION EXERCISES

When muscles aren't exercised they lose strength and mass, and if a joint isn't used it stiffens up; the aim of range-of-motion exercises is to keep your muscles and joints as strong and flexible as possible.

Here are some simple range-of-motion exercises that you can do daily. Always perform them slowly and if you feel pain, stop.

Neck and head

You can do this sitting or standing, but make sure your posture is good with your back straight and tummy tucked in.

1. Slowly turn your head to the left and look over your left shoulder as far as you can without straining, then slowly bring your head back to the centre. Repeat to the right. Do both directions 5 times, increasing your range as your neck loosens up. Remember to do this slowly, don't push your head beyond what feels comfortable and stop if you feel any pain.
2. Slowly lower your chin to your chest and let the weight of your head stretch the back of your neck. Count for 5, then raise your head again. Do this 3 times.
   Note: Don't tilt your head back as this can lead to a pinched nerve in your neck. It is best to consult your physiotherapist to see if tilting your head back is an appropriate exercise for you. If so then you can add it at this point.
3. Without turning your head or lifting your shoulders, slowly tilt your head to the left as if you were putting

your ear on your shoulder. Raise your head and do the same on the right. Repeat 3–5 times.

Shoulders and arms

Stand with your feet slightly apart, directly under your hips. Stand tall with your back straight, tummy and buttocks tucked in, arms by your sides.

1. Slowly raise your left arm until it is pointing to the ceiling. Now, slowly drop your hand until it's touching the back of your neck, or even lower if you can manage it. Clasp your elbow with your right hand and feel the stretch through your upper arm. Slowly reverse the process and bring your arm back down by your side, then continue it back and place your arm across the small of your back. Return to the starting position. Repeat with your right arm. Repeat both sides 3–5 times.
2. Start with your arms by your sides. Now slowly raise your left arm out sideways as high as it will go. Repeat 5 times. Repeat with your right arm.
3. Hold your arms out slightly from your body and begin to make small circles with them, keeping your arms straight. You can do this one arm at a time or both together, whichever feels most comfortable. Slowly increase the size of the circles until the circle is almost vertical (or as high as you can go). Slowly decrease the size again until your arms are by your sides. Repeat, changing the direction of the circle.

Hands and fingers

You can do these sitting or standing.

1. Hold your hands out in front of you with your palms facing down. Stretch your fingers out as far as they will go, then make a fist. Rest your hands for a short while, then repeat. Do this 5–10 times.
2. Hold your hands out with the palms up. Now move your thumb across your palm as if trying to touch the other

side, then back out as wide as it will go. Repeat 5–10 times.

3. Touch the tip of your little finger with the tip of your thumb, then touch all your finger tips in turn with your thumb. Repeat each set 10 times with each hand.

Legs and hips

1. Stand holding onto the back of a solid chair with one hand. Keeping your leg straight, slowly bring one leg forward until it is about 30 cm off the ground (or as high as you feel comfortable with) without leaning back. Now take it back as far as it will comfortably go without bending forward. Repeat 5 times. Repeat with your other leg.

2. (Don't do this exercise if you have had a hip replacement without discussing it with your doctor first.) In the same starting position, lift your left leg out to the side as high as it will comfortably go, then bring it back to the ground again. Repeat 3–5 times. Repeat with your other leg.

3. (Don't do this exercise if you have had a hip replacement without discussing it with your doctor first.) In the same starting position, lift your leg out to the side and make small circles with your leg, 5–10 times one way, then 5–10 times the other way. Repeat with the other leg.

4. Lie on the floor or on a firm bed. Bring your left knee up to your chest as high as it will go, then slowly lower it to the floor. Repeat 2–3 times. Repeat with the right leg.

Back and waist

1. Stand tall with your back straight, tummy and buttocks tucked in, feet parallel and about 30 cm apart. Raise your left arm at right angles to your shoulder with your palm facing right. Don't flex your hand, just let it relax. Keeping your feet still, slowly turn to your left, following your hand with your head and eyes, as far as you can go. Don't strain. Slowly return to the starting position. Repeat 2–3 times, taking your time with each turn. You will find that you can turn a little further each time, but it is

important not to strain. Repeat with the right arm, turning to the right.

2. Stand tall with your back straight, tummy and buttocks tucked in, feet parallel and about 30 cm apart. Raise your left arm and place your hand behind your head. Slowly slide your right hand down your right thigh as far as you can go. Do not strain. Feel the stretch up your left side. Return to the starting position. Repeat 3 times. Repeat on the other side.

3. Stand tall with your back straight, tummy and buttocks tucked in, feet parallel and about 30 cm apart. Bend your knees slightly and slowly roll your hips to the right, then to the back, then to the left and then the front. Do this slow circular motion 3 times in one direction and then 3 times in the other direction.

To help you get the most from these exercises:

- try to do them every day
- do them slowly
- remember to breathe as you exercise
- stop exercising if you feel any pain.

OVERDOING IT

Having extolled the virtues of exercise for arthritis I have to point out that it is possible to overdo it. Excessive exercise can cause pain and swelling of your joints, which does more harm than good. The notion of 'no pain, no gain' is completely false. As mentioned before, if joint pain persists for more than two hours after exercise, then you've done too much. You have to learn a balance and the best way to do this is to tune in to your energy levels and not overdo things. If any exercise hurts you, stop it. If you get tired, rest. Cease any exercise if you experience the following:

- dizziness
- nausea
- shortness of breath
- chest pain.

If these symptoms occur, see your doctor. To avoid overdoing it, start exercises slowly, repeat only a few times, then build up the frequency gradually.

Do range-of-motion exercises slowly and smoothly, without any jerking or bouncing. You'll get more benefit if you do them slowly and thoroughly, than if you do more of them less well. And remember, do the exercise until you feel a slight stretch, but don't force the position.

SEVEN STRATEGIES TO KEEP YOU MOTIVATED TO EXERCISE

Many of us find exercising a bit of a bore and even though we might embark on a program with enthusiasm, we soon start to find excuses not to continue. Here are some ways to keep you motivated:

1. *If you get bored*
   Use a Walkman to listen to music that you really enjoy that is happy and upbeat, or listen to the radio while you exercise. Exercise with a friend—the exercise period will soon pass in good conversation. Vary the time and location of your exercise.
2. *If the weather is bad*
   Change outdoor activity for indoor exercise like using an exercise video suitable for arthritis patients (ask the Arthritis Foundation about their tapes), go to an indoor swimming pool, join a gentle 'tone' aquarobics class, go dancing if you enjoy it. Or go for your walk inside a shopping mall!
3. *If your arthritis is active*
   You should certainly cut back on exercise during a flare-up, but try to do some form of gentle stretching. Try the range-of-motion and simple stretches suggested in this chapter.
4. *If you don't like exercising alone*
   Join a health club, yoga class or walking group. Or form your own walking or exercise circle with friends.

5. *If it hurts*

   Whenever exercise is mentioned in reference to arthritis you'll always hear the advice 'If it hurts, stop', but you must realise that starting any new exercise program is bound to cause mild aches and pains as your body gets used to unaccustomed activity. The guidelines here are to warm up with some gentle stretching for about 5 minutes before you exercise and warm down with another 5 minutes of gentle stretches at the end. Keep focused on the knowledge that exercise helps build strong muscles and joints and will ultimately reduce arthritic pain.

6. *If you feel too unfit to exercise*

   This is a bit like cleaning your house before the cleaner comes! Just because a lot of fit people parade themselves in the gym or in the park, doesn't mean less fit people shouldn't exercise. You don't have to wear figure-hugging Lycra and have a 'body beautiful' to get out there and exercise. Forget about other people. Put on comfortable clothes, get yourself good, supportive footwear and have fun. Remember your body is a willing partner in exercise and will respond well to any appropriate exercise you give it. Start slowly and build up, as discussed previously.

7. *If you are too busy to exercise*

   It only takes about 10 minutes a day doing range-of-motion exercises, and 30 minutes general exercise 3 times a week to improve your overall health and fitness—not a great deal of time to invest in your health to reduce pain, stiffness and fatigue? Try to build these times into your week and use the chart in this chapter to keep a record. Keeping a record and focusing on the goals you want to achieve can motivate you to find the time needed for exercise.

Remember, exercise will improve your overall health and fitness, reduce pain, help you sleep better, lift depression and promote a sense of well-being. It's worth it, don't you think?

9

Diet and arthritis

Can what you eat affect your arthritis? Well, that depends on who you talk to. The medical profession, in general, claims that gout is the only form of the disease with a food connection. On the other hand, western and Chinese herbal medicine practitioners believe food has a lot to do with arthritis, especially the autoimmune forms such as rheumatoid arthritis, which they think can be related to allergies. Some natural therapists recommend avoiding cheese, milk and capsicum because they believe these foods can aggravate the disease. And how many times have you been offered advice by well-meaning colleagues and friends about this or that 'food cure'? It's a mine-field of conflicting information.

So who is right? Well, although most conventional medical practitioners pooh-pooh the idea of food as medicine because, they say, there has been little scientific testing in this area, research *is* being done into the links between food and health, and the results are quite surprising. For example, in March 1997 the results of long running research from Harvard Medical School revealed that tomatoes and tomato-based products can help protect men from prostate cancer. And it is now accepted, even by mainstream health authorities, that including oily fish which contains Omega-3 fatty acids in our diet protects us against heart disease and has an anti-inflammatory effect in arthritis. So, I'm keeping an open mind—maybe these long-held beliefs by alternative medical practitioners have some validity after all. However, until the jury comes back with a positive verdict I'm still going to take my conventional medicine and recommend that you do too.

Some of you may have followed advice to eat or avoid certain foods and found that your condition has improved, but it's important to realise that arthritis can go into remission, which means that symptoms do sometimes subside for no apparent reason. Your improvement may also be due to the 'placebo effect', a recognised phenomenon whereby if you truly believe something will help, then it probably will—for a short time, at least.

My advice is to never let a 'fad diet' take the place of your medication. Adapt your diet if you believe it will help, but make sure you are still eating well and with as much variety as possible to avoid nutritional deficiencies, which will definitely not help your arthritis!

Of course, if you suffer from gout, you should watch your intake of certain foods like alcohol and offal meats such as brains, liver and sweetbreads which can aggravate this condition. However, modern medications can effectively treat and control gout now, so attention to diet is not as crucial as it once was.

One thing is certain, however, and that is eating a well-balanced diet based on the five food groups (see page 90), restricting your intake of saturated fats, salt and sugar and eating plenty of vegetables, grain foods and fruits every day will put you in the best possible condition for coping with your arthritis. It's also important to have an adequate calcium intake throughout your life to protect against osteoporosis, which is the main cause of fractures in older people (see Osteoporosis, page 79).

OSTEOPOROSIS

Osteoporosis is a condition in which bone becomes less dense, more brittle and develops a tendency to fracture easily. It's linked with the decline in production of the female sex hormone oestrogen as we age—lack of oestrogen leads to reduced absorption of calcium from foods and an increased breakdown of calcium from bone. It affects more women than men (who generally develop the disease at a later age than women) due to the drop in oestrogen that women experience after the menopause—by the age of 70 years a woman's bone density has reduced by about a third.

There are no obvious symptoms of osteoporosis, which is usually detected in bone scans and X-rays after a fracture has occurred. Your risk of developing this condition is increased if:

- your alcohol consumption is higher than the recommended safe level of two standard drinks a day for women and two–four standard drinks a day for men
- you smoke
- if you undergo prolonged treatment with corticosteroid drugs (such as those used to treat some forms of arthritis)
- you have your ovaries removed
- your diet is deficient in calcium
- you lead a sedentary life
- you suffer chronic bronchitis or emphysema.

However, there are ways of preventing or slowing down the loss of bone. Hormone replacement therapy, adequate calcium in your diet and regular weight bearing exercise (at least two brisk 30 minute walks a week) will help to keep bones strong and healthy.

Approximate daily calcium requirements

Babies	0–6	months	breast fed		formula fed
			300	mg	500 mg
	7–12	months	550	mg	
Children	1–3	years	700	mg	
	4–7	years	800	mg	
	8–11	years	800–900	mg	
	12–15	years	1000–1200	mg	
	16–18	years	800–1000	mg	
Women	19–54	years	800	mg	
	55	plus	1000	mg	
Men	19	plus	800	mg	

Foods rich in calcium include

- Milk
  whole = 230 mg per 200 ml
  skim/non fat = 240 mg per 200 ml
- Cheese
  Cheddar = 240 per 30 g
  Camembert = 150 per 30 g
- Yoghurt
  plain, including low-fat varieties = 350 per 200 g
- Canned fish with edible bones
  sardines = 350 mg per 100 g
  salmon = 190 mg per 100 g
- Vegetables
  silverbeet, cooked = 100 mg per 1/2 cup
  spinach, cooked = 100 mg per 1/2 cup
  broccoli, cooked = 50 mg per 1 cup
- Pulses
  soy beans, cooked = 90 mg per 1/2 cup
  chick peas, cooked = 75 mg per 1/2 cup
  baked beans = 60 mg per 1/2 cup
  kidney beans, cooked = 60 mg per 1/2 cup
  butter beans, cooked = 60 mg per 1/2 cup
- Nuts and seeds

> sesame seeds = 115 mg per 1 tablespoon
> almonds = 70 mg per 30 g
> Brazil nuts = 55 mg per 30 g
> pistachios = 40 mg per 30 g
> walnuts = 30 mg per 30 g
> - Miscellaneous
>   rhubarb, cooked = 170 mg per 1/2 cup
>   ice-cream = 65 mg per 1 large scoop
>   tofu = 130 mg per 1/2 cup

WEIGHT CONTROL

It's really important you keep your weight under control if you are suffering from any form of arthritis—especially osteoarthritis—to avoid placing extra stress on weight bearing

Healthy eating pyramid

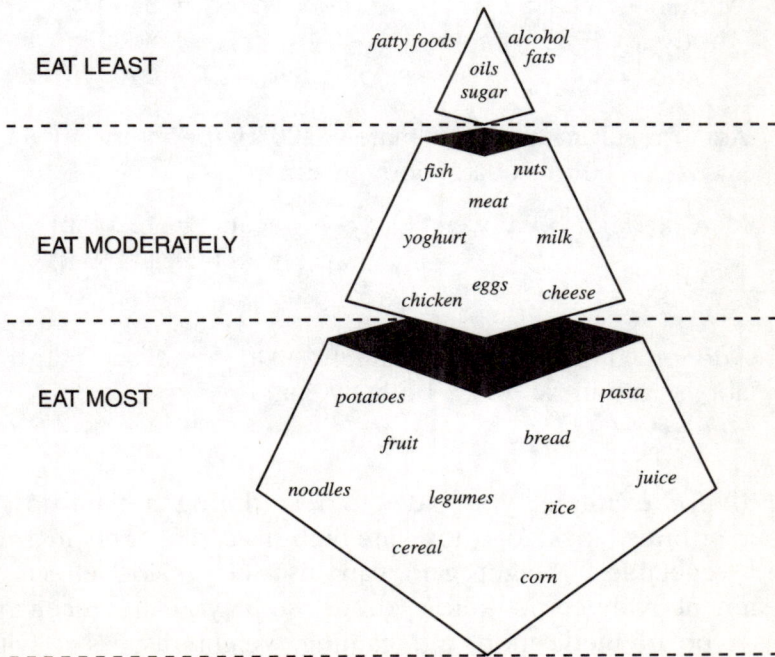

EAT LEAST

fatty foods / alcohol fats
oils
sugar

EAT MODERATELY

fish   nuts
meat
yoghurt   milk
chicken   eggs   cheese

EAT MOST

potatoes   pasta
fruit   bread
noodles   juice
legumes   rice
cereal
corn

joints such as your hips, knees and lower back. As your joints are already stressed with arthritis this is a burden they can do without.

Many people, especially if they are suffering from osteo-arthritis, have gained great relief or remission from the pain and swelling in their joints simply by slimming down.

Weight gain can occur for reasons other than simply poor dietary habits. When joints become stiff and painful you may not feel like exercising as much as you did before, and may decrease your overall activity, without adjusting your energy intake. Eating as you normally do but expending less energy will lead to weight gain, and the weight will be harder for you to lose because of your reduced activity. So watch your kilojoule intake and adjust it accordingly.

Average daily energy consumption to maintain mean body weight

Women of 60 kg body weight	18–35 years	= 8400 kJ
	6–54 years	= 7600 kJ
	55 plus	= 6400 kJ

Add or subtract approximately 400 kJ for every 5 kg above or below 60 kg body weight.

Men of 75 kg body weight	18–35 years	= 12200 kJ
	36–54 years	= 11150 kJ
	55 plus	= 9425 kJ

Add or subtract approximately 600 kJ for every 5 kg above or below 75 kg body weight.

If, for example, you have to rest during a flare-up of your arthritis, stick to a low-fat, high-fibre diet, rich in fruit and vegetables. Weight gain can also be a side effect of treatment with corticosteroid drugs, so if you are receiving this type of medication and gaining weight discuss it with your doctor.

Weight to height table (based on a medium frame)

Women		Men	
Height (cm)	Weight (kg)	Height (cm)	Weight (kg)
143	44–49	155	54–59
145	45–50	158	55–60
148	46–51	160	56–62
150	47–53	163	58–63
153	49–54	165	59–65
155	50–55	168	61–67
158	51–57	170	63–69
160	53–59	173	64–71
163	54–61	175	66–73
165	56–63	178	68–75
168	58–65	180	70–77
170	60–67	183	72–79
173	62–69	185	74–82
175	63–70	188	76–84
178	65–72	190	78–86
180	67–74	193	80–88

EFFECTIVE WEIGHT LOSS THROUGH DIETARY FAT REDUCTION

For effective weight loss it is important to count grams of fat rather than kilojoules, as it has been shown that reducing fats is the single most important factor for weight reduction (see Fat—the good and the bad).

FAT—THE GOOD AND THE BAD

It's important for good nutrition to understand the role that fat plays in our well-being. We all need some fat in our diet to provide the essential fatty acids and fat-soluble vitamins—A, D, E and K—required for good health. However, there are good and bad fats and which ones we choose to eat can make all the difference to our health. There are three main types of fat—saturated, monounsaturated and polyunsaturated—and foods containing fat will usually have all three but with one type predominating.

The good—polyunsaturated and monounsaturated fats

It's recommended that no more than 25 per cent of kilojoule intake should come from fat and this should come from the polyunsaturated or monounsaturated types.

Polyunsaturated fats are mainly found in vegetable oils (such as corn, safflower, sunflower, walnut and soya bean oils), nuts, cereals and oily fish such as sardines, mackerel, tuna and salmon.

Monounsaturated fats are found in foods such as olives and olive oil, canola oil, macadamia nuts and oil, peanuts and peanut oil, and avocados.

The bad—saturated fats

Found in fatty meats, full-cream dairy products, dripping, margarine, cooking fats, etc., saturated fat has been shown to raise blood cholesterol levels. A high cholesterol level is one of the major factors linked to the development of heart disease, as well as contributing to overweight and obesity. (See below for ways to reduce the fat in your diet.)

To reduce fat in your diet to about 25 per cent of kilojoule intake would mean consuming 30–40 g of fat per day for women and 40–60 g of fat for men. Obvious fat, like butter (which contains 5 g of fat in every teaspoon), the fat on meat and skin on chicken, is easy to avoid, but there's a great deal of 'hidden' fat in processed and manufactured food, so read the labels to see how much fat there is per serve, or buy one of the handy, pocket-size fat counters that are on the market. You'll be amazed to see just how much fat you consume each day.

Here are some easy ways to help reduce fat in your diet:

• Use low-fat foods such as lean meat trimmed of all fat, chicken with the skin removed, skim milk and low-fat cheeses.

- Avoid fried foods, pastries, 'deli' meats, snack foods, rich cakes and biscuits.
- Choose low-fat take-away foods such as salad sandwiches or rolls, fruit, barbecued chicken (without skin) and lean hamburgers (without fried egg) with lots of salad, fruit salads, etc.
- Cook using low-fat methods, such as grilling, steaming, baking and stir frying.
- Use low-fat cottage cheese, ricotta or avocado as a sandwich spread, or spread polyunsaturated margarine very thinly.
- Skim fat from the tops of soups and casseroles.
- Avoid battered or crumbed foods.
- Use low-fat yoghurt, lemon juice or vinegar instead of mayonnaise or salad oils.

If you are unsure of how to go about successfully losing weight, then ask your doctor to refer you to a dietitian for advice.

Fat, fibre and carbohydrate content for food

Note: Figures can only be approximate as food samples can vary with the season, degree of freshness and place of origin.

Food	Fat (g)	Fibre (g)	Carbohydrate (g)
Breads			
Bread			
white, 2 slices	2	2	27
wholemeal, 2 slices	2	4	23
mixed grain, 2 slices	1	3	27
Croissant, one	19	1	28
Crumpet, one	1	1.5	24
Damper, 50 g piece	5	1	38
Danish pastry, one	15	1	38
Doughnut (plain), one	10	0.5	25
Muffin			
American-style, one	2	0	7
English-style, one	1	2	31
Pita, 50 g piece	1	2	29
Dairy products			
Buttermilk, 250 mL	2	0	11
Condensed milk, 20 mL	2	0	11
Cow's milk, 250 mL	10	0	12
Cream, 20 mL	10	0	0.5
Evaporated milk, 125 mL	11	0	14
Skim milk, 250 mL	0	0	12

Food	Fat (g)	Fibre (g)	Carbohydrate (g)
Yoghurt, (plain) 200 g	8	0	12
Cheese			
Blue, 30 g	9	0	0
Brie, 30 g	9	0	0
Camembert, 30 g	8	0	0
Cheddar, 30 g	11	0	0
Colby, 30 g	11	0	0
Cottage cheese, 30 g	2	0	0
Cotto, 30 g	3	0	0
Cream cheese, 30 g	15	0	0
Edam, 30 g	8	0	0
Fetta (reduced fat), 30 g	5	0	0
Gouda, 30 g	9	0	0
Havarti, 30 g	11	0	0
Mozzarella, 30 g	7	0	0
Parmesan, 30 g	10	0	0
Ricotta, 30 g	4	0	0
Swiss, 30 g	9	0	0
Cereals and cereal products			
Barley (cooked) 1/2 cup	1	5	35
Buckwheat (cooked), 50 g	1	6	36
Oats (rolled, cooked), 1/2 cup	1	1	81
Rice			
brown (cooked), 1/2 cup	1	2	38
calrose (cooked), 1/2 cup	neg.	neg.	17
white (cooked) 1/2 cup	neg.	neg.	39
Couscous (steamed), 100 g	1	0	51
Wheatgerm, 10 g	1	2	3
Pasta (egg, cooked), 100 g	3	4	61
Noodles			
rice (cooked), 100 g	0	0	81
wheat (cooked), 100 g	6	5	75
Fresh fruit			
Apple, 125 g	0	2	17
Apricot, 100 g	0	3	11
Banana, 100 g	0	4	2
Cherries, 100 g	0	2	12
Dates, 50 g	0	13	38
Figs, 100 g	0	3	8
Grapes, 100 g	0	3	17
Grapefruit, 100 g	0	3	5
Melon, 100 g	0	1	6
Kiwifruit, 100 g	0	3	10
Lemon, 50 g	0	2	1
Lime, 50 g	0	2	1
Lychee, 100 g	0	1	16
Mandarin, 100 g	0	28	8
Mango, 100 g	0	2	15
Nectarine, 100 g	0	3	8
Orange, 200 g	0	4	11
Passionfruit, 30 g	0	4	3
Pawpaw, 100 g	0	2	7
Peach, 200 g	0	4	12
Pear, 200 g	0	5	19
Pineapple, 100 g	0	3	11

Food	Fat (g)	Fibre (g)	Carbohydrate (g)
Plum, 100 g	0	2	10
Raspberry, 100 g	0	8	6
Strawberry, 100 g	0	2	3
Tomato, 100 g	0	2	3
Watermelon, 100 g	0	0.5	5
Vegetables			
Alfalfa sprouts (raw) 15 g	0	neg.	0
Asparagus (cooked), 100 g	0	2	0
Avocado (raw), 100 g	24 g	2	0
Artichoke (globe, edible parts), 100 g	0	4	3
Artichoke (Jerusalem), 100 g	0	3	3
Bamboo shoots, 50 g	0	1	3
Beans, broad (fresh) 125 g	0	5	9
Beans, green (fresh) 50 g	0	2	3
Beetroot (cooked), 30 g	0	0.5	2
Broccoli (cooked), 50 g	0	3	1
Brussels sprouts (cooked), 100 g	0	4	4
Cabbage (raw) 50 g	0	1	3
Capsicum (raw) 100 g	0	2	7
Carrot (raw) 50 g	0	2	4
Cauliflower (steamed), 50 g	0	2	3
Celery (raw), 50 g	0	1	2
Cucumber (raw), 50 g	0	0.5	2
Eggplant (grilled), 100 g	0	3	3
Leeks (steamed), 50 g	0	2	3
Lettuce (raw), 30 g	0	0.5	2
Mushrooms (raw), 50 g	0	2	0
Onion (raw), 100 g	0	1	5
Parsnip (steamed), 100 g	0	3	15
Peas (raw), 100 g	0	5	10
Potatoes (boiled with skin), 150 g	0	2	28
Silverbeet (steamed), 50 g	0	2	3
Squash (steamed), 50 g	0	1	1
Sweet corn (boiled), 150 g	0	6	28
Sweet potato (steamed), 150 g	0	3	50
Turnip (steamed), 100 g	0	3	5
Zucchini (steamed), 50 g	0	1	1
Meat (lean cuts and poultry)			
Beef (rump, trimmed, grilled), 100 g	9	0	0
Lamb (leg, trimmed, roasted), 100 g	7	0	0
Pork (leg steak, grilled), 100 g	3	0	0
Veal (loin, trimmed, grilled), 100 g	4	0	0
Goat (leg, trimmed, roasted), 100 g	9	0	0
Kangaroo (fillet, grilled), 100 g	4	0	0
Rabbit (lean meat only), 100 g	4	0	0
Venison (leg, roasted), 100 g	6	0	0
Chicken (breast, roasted, no skin), 100 g	4	0	0
Eggs, one, 50 g	5	0	0
Duck (roasted, no skin), 100 g	10	0	0
Goose (breast, roasted, no skin), 100 g	22	0	0
Turkey (breast, roasted, no skin), 100 g	2	0	0
Deli meats			
Bacon (grilled), 50 g	6	0	0
Bratwurst (grilled), 100 g	32	0	0

Food	Fat (g)	Fibre (g)	Carbohydrate (g)
Cabanossi, 50 g	15	0	0
Chicken roll, 50 g	3	0	0
Chorizo, 100 g	30	0	0
Corned beef, 50 g	3	0	0
Devon, 50 g	8	0	0
Frankfurter, 100 g	20	0	0
Ham (leg), 50 g	3	0	0
Knackwurst, 100 g	33	0	0
Kransky, 100 g	33	0	0
Liverwurst (pork), 25 g	7	0	0
Mortadella, 50 g	15	0	0
Pancetta, 25 g	16	0	0
Pastrami, 25 g	16	0	0
Pate, 25 g	6	0	0
Salami, 50 g	18	0	0
Sausages (fresh):			
Beef (grilled), 100 g	17	0	0
Pork (grilled), 100 g	25	0	0
Chipolata (grilled), 100 g	24	0	0
Chicken (grilled), 100 g	12	0	0
Fresh fish (fat content may vary from season to season)			
Barramundi (grilled), 100 g	2	0	0
Bream (grilled), 100 g	2	0	0
Coral trout (grilled), 100 g	2	0	0
Dory (grilled), 100 g	1	0	0
Emperor (grilled), 100 g	2	0	0
Flathead (grilled), 100 g	2	0	0
Gemfish (grilled), 100 g	2	0	0
Herring (grilled), 100 g	18	0	0
Jewfish (grilled), 100 g	2	0	0
Kingfish (grilled), 100 g	3	0	0
Ling (grilled), 100 g	2	0	0
Mackerel (grilled), 100 g	16	0	0
Mullet (grilled), 100 g	7	0	0
Orange roughy (grilled), 100 g	2	0	0
Salmon (grilled), 100 g	12	0	0
Sardine (grilled), 100 g	9	0	0
Shark (grilled), 100 g	1	0	0
Snapper (grilled), 100 g	1	0	0
Trout (grilled), 100 g	5	0	0
Tuna (grilled), 100 g	3	0	0
Whiting (grilled), 100 g	1	0	0
Shellfish			
Abalone (steamed) 100 g	2	0	5
Clams (steamed), 100 g	2	0	1
Crab (boiled), 100 g	5	0	0
Mussels (steamed), 100 g	2	0	0
Octopus (barbecued), 100 g	1	0	0
Oysters (natural), 100 g	1	0	0
Prawns (boiled), 100 g	2	0	0
Scallops (steamed), 100 g	1	0	0
Squid (barbecued), 100 g	1	0	0
Yabbie (boiled), 100 g	1	0	1
Canned fish			
Anchovies (canned), 3 fillets	2	0	0

Food	Fat (g)	Fibre (g)	Carbohydrate (g)
Salmon (red, canned), 100 g	12	0	0
Sardines (canned in oil), 100 g	16	0	0
Shrimps (canned), 100 g	2	0	0
Tuna (canned in oil), 100 g	10	0	0
(canned in brine), 100 g	3	0	0
Fats and oils			
Almond oil, 20 mL	20	0	0
Avocado oil, 20 mL	20	0	0
Butter, 20 g	17	0	0
Coconut oil, 20 mL	20	0	0
Corn oil, 20 mL	20	0	0
Dripping, 20 g	20	0	0
Ghee, 20 g	20	0	0
Grapeseed oil, 20 mL	20	0	0
Hazelnut oil, 20 mL	20	0	0
Lard, 20 g	20	0	0
Macadamia oil, 20 mL	20	0	0
Margarine (table), 20 g	16	0	0
Olive oil, 20 mL	20	0	0
Peanut oil, 20 mL	20	0	0
Safflower oil, 20 mL	20	0	0
Sesame oil, 20 mL	20	0	0
Sunflower oil, 20 mL	20	0	0
Walnut oil, 20 mL	20	0	0
Nuts			
Almonds, 30 g	16	5	1
Brazil nuts, 30 g	18	3	1
Cashew nuts, 30 g	14	2	8
Chestnuts, 100 g	3	7	37
Coconut, 30 g	10	4	2
Hazelnuts, 30 g	11	2	2
Macadamias, 30 g	20	7	2
Peanuts (roasted), 30 g	15	3	3
Pecan nuts, 30 g	22	3	4
Pinenuts, 30 g	18	3	5
Pistachio nuts, 30 g	16	3	5
Walnuts, 30 g	15	2	2
Miscellaneous foods			
Baked beans (canned), 200 g	1	10	20
Dried beans (haricot, cooked), 200 g	1	15	33
Canned fruit (average), 100 g	0	1	25
Peanut butter, 25 g	12	2	3
Potato crisps (traditional), 25 g	7	1	12
Spaghetti (canned), 200 g	1	0	24
Pizza, 150 g wedge	16	3	40
Sausage roll, 150 g	26	2	40
Meat pie, 150 g	22	2	30
Pastry			
Puff, 50 g	20	1	23
Shortcrust, 50 g	20	1	27
Filo, 50 g	1	2	35

PLAN FOR HEALTHY EATING

Even if you are not overweight, it's still important to cut down on saturated fats and eat a variety of foods from the five food groups. These groups are: breads and cereals; fruit and vegetables; meat, fish, poultry, eggs, nuts and legumes; dairy products; fats and oils. See 'Healthy eating pyramid' page 81.

Breads and cereals

This group includes fibre-enriched white, multigrain and wholemeal breads; cereals such as rice, oats and rye; pasta. These foods provide energy, carbohydrate, fibre and B group vitamins. You should aim to have four or more servings a day with one serving equivalent to one slice of bread, half a cup of cooked rice or pasta or 1 cup breakfast cereal.

Fruit and vegetables

These foods not only provide carbohydrate and fibre but also B group vitamins, vitamins C and E, beta carotene (a powerful antioxidant) and potassium. Eat four or more servings a day, including one rich in vitamin C such as oranges, tomatoes, capsicum etc.

Meat, fish, poultry, eggs, nuts and legumes

This is the protein group which provides B group vitamins, including vitamin B_{12}, and vital minerals such as iron and zinc. Include one or two servings. One serving would be equivalent to 100 g cooked lean meat, fish or poultry, 1 egg, 1/4 cup raw nuts or 1/2–1 cup cooked peas, beans or lentils.

Dairy products

Try to choose low-fat varieties of products such as milk, cheeses, yoghurt etc. Adults up to about the age of 54 need 800 mg of milk each day or its equivalent to provide enough calcium and riboflavin in their diet. Women over that age need about 1000 mg (see 'Osteoporosis' page 79).

Fats and oils

Try to keep these to a minimum and remember that fat exists in many foods even though you may not be able to see it.

PUTTING IT ALL TOGETHER

The following will give you an idea of how to incorporate the principles of eating from the five food groups into your daily meals.

Breakfast

1/2–1 cup of wholegrain breakfast cereal, muesli or porridge (unsweetened), topped with a sliced banana, canned peaches or fresh berries, with skim or low-fat milk; 1–2 slices wholegrain toast topped with melted, low-fat or reduced-fat cheese, baked beans, grilled tomato or mushrooms, or a poached egg.

Lunch

2 slices of multigrain bread with low-fat filling and salad. One piece of fruit or a fruit juice. When making sandwiches, there are many ingredients which make good alternative spreads to butter or margarine. If you're having a beef sandwich, for instance, spread one slice of bread with English mustard and the other slice with horseradish, then fill with lean beef and salad; for lamb, try mint jelly and grain mustard; for chicken try cranberry sauce and a little avocado; for pork, try apple sauce and mango chutney. The list of combinations is only limited by your imagination!

Evening meal

Lean meat, fish, peas or beans, accompanied by pasta, rice, potato or bread, steamed vegetables or salad (see recipes).

If you do get hungry during the day then you can snack on wholemeal crispbreads, rice cakes, vegetable juices, fruit and low-fat yoghurt.

Aim to:

- eat a varied diet which includes foods rich in vitamins and minerals, especially iron and calcium
- reduce saturated animal fats in your diet
- include high-fibre foods and drink plenty of water as well
- eat fish two or three times a week
- get your weight down to the normal weight range, then maintain it.

10

Low-fat recipes

People always imagine that a low-fat diet is tasteless and unsatisfying, lacking the flavour which butter, cheese and cream can impart to a meal. But that simply isn't the case. Using wonderful, fresh ingredients and simplified cooking techniques, you can prepare truly delicious meals and not really be aware that they are low in fat. Here are some low-fat recipes to get you started.

MAIN MEAL SALADS

CHICKEN CAESAR SALAD

    1 tablespoon dried Italian herbs
    4 chicken breast fillets, trimmed of any skin or fat
    1 cos lettuce, washed and dried thoroughly
    1 punnet cherry tomatoes, halved
    3/4 cup bread croutons, dry toasted in the oven
    2 tablespoons grated parmesan cheese
    Dressing
    1 anchovy fillet, mashed
    1 teaspoon grain mustard
    freshly ground black pepper to taste
    1 clove garlic, crushed

1/2 cup low-fat buttermilk
1 tablespoon lemon juice
1/4 teaspoon Worcestershire sauce

1. Sprinkle Italian dried herbs over chicken. Grill or barbecue for about 5 minutes each side or until cooked through. Set aside and slice when cool.
2. Mash anchovy fillet with mustard, pepper and garlic. Stir in buttermilk, lemon juice and Worcestershire sauce. Mix well until combined.
3. Place the lettuce into a bowl. Pour dressing over. Toss well. Divide lettuce between serving plates. Scatter tomatoes and croutons over. Top with sliced chicken. Serve sprinkled with parmesan cheese.

Serves 4

CHAR-GRILLED STEAK SALAD

500 g rump steak, trimmed of all fat
1 tablespoon cracked black pepper
mixed salad leaves
1 punnet cherry tomatoes
425 g can baby corn, drained
1 tablespoon toasted sesame seeds
Dressing
2 tablespoons salt-reduced soy sauce
2 tablespoons balsamic vinegar
2 teaspoons brown sugar
1 teaspoon sesame oil
1 teaspoon freshly chopped ginger
2 cloves garlic, crushed

1. Press the cracked black pepper firmly onto both sides of the steak. Char-grill or barbecue the steak until done to taste. Set aside and slice when cool.
2. Combine dressing ingredients.
3. Place the salad leaves into a bowl. Pour dressing over. Toss well. Divide leaves among serving plates. Top with

tomatoes, corn and sliced steak and a sprinkling of toasted sesame seeds.

Serves 4

MANGO SALSA

Use this delicious salsa with lean cooked chicken breast or lean pork and serve with mixed salad leaves.

1 large ripe mango, stoned, peeled and diced
1/2 small red capsicum, seeded and finely chopped
1/2 small yellow capsicum, seeded and finely chopped
1/2 small red onion, very finely chopped
1 clove garlic, minced
2 tablespoons balsamic vinegar
2 tablespoons chopped fresh coriander
freshly ground black pepper to taste

Combine all ingredients. Cover and refrigerate for at least an hour before serving over lean, cold meats and salad.
Makes about 2 cups

DRESSINGS FOR SALADS

LEMON CUCUMBER DRESSING

200 g non-fat skim milk yoghurt
1 cucumber, peeled, seeded and chopped
1 clove garlic, crushed
1 tablespoon freshly squeezed lemon juice
1 tablespoon finely chopped fresh parsley
1/2 teaspoon grated lemon peel
freshly ground black pepper to taste

Combine all ingredients. Refrigerate until ready to serve.
Makes 1 cup

TARRAGON MUSTARD DRESSING

1/4 cup non-fat skim milk yoghurt
2 tablespoons freshly squeezed lemon juice

1 tablespoon French mustard
1/2 teaspoon dried tarragon
freshly ground black pepper to taste

Combine all ingredients. Refrigerate until ready to serve.
Makes 1/2 cup

TOMATO HORSERADISH DRESSING

1/2 cup pureed tomatoes
2 tablespoons prepared horseradish
2 teaspoons white wine vinegar
1 teaspoon salt-reduced soy sauce
1 teaspoon dry mustard
pinch ground nutmeg
pinch ground cloves

Combine all ingredients. Refrigerate until ready to use.
Makes 3/4 cup

CHICKEN DISHES

CHICKEN AND SESAME STIR FRY

1/4 cup chicken stock
2 large chicken breast fillets, trimmed of any skin or fat
and cut into strips
1 carrot, chopped
1 stick celery, chopped
2 shallots, chopped
1 tablespoon soy sauce
1 teaspoon honey
1 tablespoon sesame seeds

1. Place 1 tablespoon chicken stock in a non-stick wok over
high heat. Stir fry chicken strips for 3–4 minutes. Remove
from pan with a slotted spoon.
2. Add another tablespoon chicken stock to wok and stir
fry carrot, celery and shallots for 2–3 minutes.
3. Return chicken to pan with remaining stock, soy sauce

and honey. Stir fry a further 2 minutes. Sprinkle over sesame seeds and serve over plain boiled rice or noodles.

Serves 4

MARMALADE MUSTARD CHICKEN

1/2 cup marmalade
1/4 cup French mustard
1/2 tablespoon freshly squeezed lemon juice
4 large chicken breast fillets, trimmed of any skin or fat

1. Melt marmalade in a small saucepan over gentle heat. Blend in mustard and lemon juice. Cool slightly.
2. Place the chicken on a foil-lined grill tray. Grill for about 2 minutes each side. Brush with marmalade baste. Continue cooking for a further 2–3 minutes each side or until cooked, basting as you turn the chicken. Watch the chicken carefully, because the sugar in the marmalade attracts heat and may scorch easily. Serve sliced in a tossed mixed salad.

Serves 4

TANDOORI CHICKEN

500 g chicken thigh fillets, trimmed of any skin or fat
1 cup non-fat skim milk yoghurt
1/4 cup prepared tandoori paste
1 tablespoon paprika
4 cups cooked long-grain rice

1. Place chicken in a casserole dish in one layer. Combine yoghurt and tandoori paste in a bowl, mix well. Pour over chicken, coat well. Cover and refrigerate overnight.
2. Preheat oven to 180°C. Sprinkle paprika over chicken. Bake for 30–40 minutes or until cooked.
3. Serve with long-grain rice, pappadams (cooked in the microwave) and sambals of cucumber and non-fat skim milk yoghurt, tomato, onion and mint, and sliced banana in lemon juice.

Serves 4

LEMON THYME CHICKEN

juice 1 lemon
few sprigs fresh lemon thyme
1/4 cup white wine
salt and freshly ground black pepper to taste
4 chicken breasts, trimmed of all skin and fat, cut into
     thick strips
extra sprigs of lemon thyme
125 g button mushrooms, sliced

1. Combine lemon juice, lemon thyme and white wine. Season to taste. Add chicken, stir well. Marinate for 1 hour.
2. Arrange chicken and extra lemon thyme in a steaming basket. Steam over boiling water for 5 minutes. Add mushrooms and continue to cook a further 4 minutes. Serve with rice and a dipping sauce of combined soy sauce, sherry and wasabi, if desired.

Serves 4

PORK DISHES

PORK FILLET IN A MUSTARD CRUST

1 1/2 cups mango chutney
1/4 cup grain mustard
500 g New Fashioned pork fillet, trimmed of any fat
1 1/2 cups wholemeal dried breadcrumbs

1. Preheat oven to 180°C. Combine 1/2 cup chutney and mustard in a small bowl. Coat pork fillet with chutney/mustard mixture, then roll in breadcrumbs to coat.
2. Place pork on a rack in a baking tray. Bake for 25–30 minutes or until cooked.
3. Stand for 10 minutes, before serving sliced with remaining mango chutney, a crisp green salad, and crusty bread.

Serves 4

BARBECUED PORK KEBABS

500 g diced New Fashioned Pork
4 yellow zucchinis, cut into 3 cm pieces
16 button mushrooms
16 small pickling onions, peeled and blanched
8 bamboo skewers, soaked in water for 30 minutes
Marinade
2 tablespoons plum sauce
2 tablespoons reduced-salt soy sauce
2 tablespoons tomato sauce
1 tablespoon white wine
1 clove garlic, finely chopped
1 tablespoon grated orange rind
1 teaspoon minced ginger
1 teaspoon sesame oil
1/2 teaspoon Chinese five spice powder

1. Combine marinade ingredients in a bowl. Pour over pork and coat well. Cover and refrigerate overnight.
2. Drain pork, reserving marinade. Thread pork, zucchinis, mushrooms and onions alternately on skewers. Brush with marinade and grill or barbecue for about 5 minutes each side until pork is cooked.

Serves 4

MOROCCAN PORK

1 1/4 cups chicken stock
1/4 cup white wine
1/2 cup orange juice
1 tablespoon minced ginger
2 cloves
sprinkling freshly grated nutmeg (optional)
500 g pork fillet, trimmed
1 large carrot, sliced diagonally
1/3 cup sultanas
2 tablespoons toasted pinenuts

1. Preheat oven to 180°C. Combine chicken stock, white wine, orange juice, ginger, cloves and nutmeg in a saucepan, bring to the boil, remove from heat.
2. Place pork in a casserole dish with the carrot and sultanas. Pour combined sauce ingredients over, cover and bake for 35–45 minutes or until pork is cooked. Remove pork and let meat stand 5 minutes. Meanwhile, reduce pan juices until slightly thickened. Serve pork sliced on top of couscous with pan juices poured over and scattered with pinenuts.

Serves 4

LAMB DISHES

BARBECUED ROSEMARY LAMB

4 Trim Lamb leg steaks
fresh mint for garnish
Marinade
1 clove garlic, crushed
1 red onion, chopped
1/4 cup white wine
2 tablespoons lemon juice
1/2 teaspoon rosemary
2 bay leaves
1 teaspoon grated lemon peel

1. Combine marinade ingredients. Pour over lamb, making sure it is well coated. Cover and refrigerate overnight.
2. Drain lamb, reserve marinade. Barbecue or char-grill lamb, basting with marinade, until cooked to taste. Garnish with fresh mint and serve with jacket potatoes and corn cobs.

Serves 4

SPICY LAMB CASSEROLE

500 g Trim Lamb leg steak, cubed
1 tablespoon chopped fresh mint

Marinade
1 cup non-fat skim milk yoghurt
1 tablespoon ground cumin
1 tablespoon ground coriander
1 tablespoon garam masala
1 teaspoon ground cardamom

1. Combine marinade ingredients in a bowl. Place lamb in a casserole dish and pour yoghurt marinade mixture over. Cover and refrigerate for at least 2 hours.
2. Preheat oven to 160°C. Bake, covered, for about 1 1/2 hours until lamb is tender. Serve with boiled long grain rice, microwaved pappadams and mango chutney.

Serves 4

GLAZED APRICOT LAMB

500 g Trim Lamb topside mini-roast
200 mL bottle apricot nectar
1/4 cup white wine
1 clove garlic, crushed
1 teaspoon dried rosemary

1. Preheat oven to 220°C. Place meat on a roasting rack in a baking pan.
2. Combine remaining ingredients and brush over the lamb, reserving a little apricot mixture.
3. Roast for 45 minutes or until lamb is cooked to taste, brushing frequently with apricot mixture.
4. Remove from oven and let stand for 10 minutes. Meanwhile combine any remaining apricot mixture with the pan juices and reduce over high heat until slightly thickened. Serve lamb sliced with baby potatoes and steamed vegetables with pan juices poured over.

Serves 4

BEEF DISHES

BEEF BURGUNDY

> 500 g lean round steak, trimmed of any fat, cubed
> 2 tablespoons plain flour, seasoned with salt and pepper
> vegetable oil spray
> 1 1/2 cups beef stock
> 1 cup burgundy wine (or other red wine as preferred)
> 1/2 teaspoon dried mixed herbs
> 1 large clove garlic, minced
> 1 large onion, cut into eighths
> 2 carrots, chopped
> 2 sticks celery, chopped
> 125 g button mushrooms
> 4 potatoes, peeled and diced
> 2 tablespoons finely chopped fresh parsley

1. Preheat oven to 260°C. Dust meat with flour. Place in a casserole dish which has been sprayed with vegetable oil. Roast for about 5 minutes, stir and roast for a further 5 minutes. Remove from oven, stand 5 minutes. Reduce heat to 180°C.
2. Pour stock and wine into casserole dish. Stir to loosen meat and any browned bits sticking to the bottom. Add mixed herbs and garlic. Bake, covered, for 1 hour. Add remaining ingredients, except parsley. Continue cooking for 20–30 minutes until the meat and vegetables are tender. Serve sprinkled with parsley.

Serves 4

BEEF STROGANOFF

> 500 g rump steak, trimmed of any fat, cut into strips
> 250 g cup mushrooms, sliced
> 1 onion, sliced
> 2 cloves garlic, crushed
> vegetable oil spray
> 1 tablespoon reduced fat, polyunsaturated margarine

2 tablespoons plain flour
1 cup beef stock
salt and pepper to taste
1/4 cup low-fat sour cream
3 cups cooked noodles, hot
finely chopped fresh parsley

1. Cook steak, mushrooms, onion and garlic in a large non-stick frying pan coated with cooking spray over medium-high heat, stirring constantly, until tender. Remove from pan with a slotted spoon. Wipe pan clean.
2. Melt margarine in pan over low heat, add flour, stir until smooth. Cook 1 minute, stirring constantly. Gradually stir in stock, stirring constantly over medium heat, until thickened. Season to taste. Add steak mixture. Cook gently until thoroughly heated.
3. Remove from heat and stir in sour cream (do not reheat). Serve over noodles, sprinkled with parsley.

Serves 4

ROAST BEEF IN RED WINE

1 carrot, cut into matchsticks
1 parsnip, cut into matchsticks
1 onion, sliced
1 stick celery, sliced
2 cloves garlic, crushed
500 g lean beef roast, trimmed
salt and pepper to taste
3/4 cup red wine
3/4 cup beef stock

1. Preheat oven to 220°C. Make a bed of the vegetables and garlic in a roasting pan and place beef on top. Season to taste with salt and pepper. Roast in the oven for 10 minutes.
2. Reduce heat to 180°C. Pour combined wine and stock over meat and mix with pan juices. Baste beef with pan juices. Continue cooking for a further 20–30 minutes or

until beef is cooked to taste, basting with pan juices from time to time.

3. Remove from oven and let stand for 10 minutes. Meanwhile, strain pan juices and reduce over high heat until slightly thickened. Serve beef sliced with vegetables and pan juices poured over.

Serves 4

SEAFOOD DISHES

SEASONED BAKED SNAPPER

1/4 cup fish or chicken stock
1/4 cup white wine
1 onion, chopped
2 cloves garlic, crushed
1 stick celery, chopped
1 tablespoon freshly squeezed lemon juice
1 tablespoon pinenuts, toasted
1 tablespoon chopped fresh parsley
1/4 cup dried breadcrumbs
1 large snapper, cleaned but head and tail left on
1/4 cup lime juice
1/4 cup tomato juice

1. Preheat oven to 180°C. Simmer stock, wine, onion, garlic and celery for 2–3 minutes or until the vegetables have softened. Add the lemon juice, pinenuts, parsley and breadcrumbs. Stir well.
2. Fill fish cavity with stuffing. Secure opening closed with a wooden or metal skewer. Place fish in baking dish. Pour combined lime juice and tomato juice over.
3. Bake, covered, for 30–40 minutes, basting frequently, until cooked. Serve fish and stuffing with pan juices spooned over. Plain baked or boiled potatoes go beautifully with this dish.

Serves 4

SCALLOPS IN COINTREAU AND ORANGE

    1 tablespoon Cointreau (or demi sec)
    grated rind 1 orange
    1/2 teaspoon fresh chopped ginger
    1/4 teaspoon ground nutmeg
    1/4 teaspoon ground cinnamon
    1/4 teaspoon ground allspice
    salt and freshly ground white pepper to taste
    500 g scallops, cleaned
    juice of 1 orange
    4 cups cooked jasmine rice

1. Combine Cointreau, orange rind, ginger, nutmeg, cinnamon and allspice in a bowl. Season to taste with salt and pepper.
2. Pour over scallops and mix well. Pour into a non-stick frying pan and gently sauté scallops until cooked, about 3 minutes.
3. Remove scallops from pan and keep warm. Add orange juice to pan and stir until sauce begins to bubble. Serve scallops over cooked jasmine rice with sauce poured over.

Serves 4

SALMON AND DILL PARCELS

    4 salmon cutlets
    1 small lemon, sliced
    1 small onion, cut into thin slices
    1 tablespoon chopped fresh dill (or 1 teaspoon dried)
    4 tablespoons white wine

1. Preheat oven to 180°C. Place each salmon cutlet on a square of foil large enough to fold round it into a secure parcel. Top each cutlet with lemon and onion slices, then sprinkle with dill and wine. Fold foil to form a secure parcel.
2. Place parcels on a baking tray and bake for 15–20 minutes or until cooked to taste.

3. Serve salmon in foil parcels with baby potatoes and steamed vegetables.

Serves 4

PASTA DISHES

PASTA PUTTANESCA

2 x 425 g cans Italian peeled tomatoes
45 g can anchovy fillets, drained and blotted dry with
  paper towel
75 g stuffed green olives, sliced
2 tablespoons capers
1 teaspoon dried Italian mixed herbs
cracked black pepper to taste
375 g dry pasta of choice

1. Place undrained tomatoes into a blender. Process until smooth. Transfer to a small saucepan. Add anchovies, olives, capers, herbs and pepper. Simmer slowly until sauce begins to thicken (time will vary depending on juiciness of tomatoes).
2. Cook pasta until al dente. Drain and place into serving bowls. Divide sauce among the bowls and serve with a green salad and crusty bread.

Serves 4

PASTA WITH BASIL AND BEANS

1 small onion, chopped
1 clove garlic, crushed
1/4 cup chicken stock
1 small yellow capsicum, chopped
1 stick celery, chopped
425 g four-bean mix, drained
425 g can peeled tomatoes
1 tablespoon chopped fresh basil
375 g dry pasta of choice

1. Sauté onion and garlic in stock for 3–4 minutes. Add capsicum, celery, beans and tomatoes and continue cooking over gentle heat for a further 10 minutes, until sauce has slightly thickened. Add basil and continue cooking for 5 more minutes.
2. Meanwhile, cook pasta until al dente. Drain and serve with bean and basil sauce.

Serves 4

PASTA PRIMAVERA

1 onion, chopped
1 clove garlic, crushed
1 large tomato, peeled, seeded and chopped
1 green capsicum, chopped
100 g mushrooms, sliced
1/4 cup chicken stock
1/4 cup no-oil Italian salad dressing
1 tablespoon chopped fresh basil
salt and pepper to taste
375 g dried pasta of choice

1. Simmer onion, garlic, tomatoes, capsicum and mushrooms in stock for 3–4 minutes or until softened. Add the salad dressing, basil, and season to taste with salt and pepper.
2. Meanwhile cook pasta until al dente. Drain and serve with sauce poured over, accompanied by crusty bread and a mixed salad.

Serves 4

DESSERTS

SHERRIED BAKED APPLES

1/2 cup sultanas
1/2 cup chopped dates
1/2 teaspoon ground cinnamon
1/4 teaspoon ground cloves
1 1/4 cups pear juice

1/4 cup sweet sherry
4 apples, cored

1. Place the sultanas, dates, cinnamon and cloves into a glass dish. Pour 1/2 cup pear juice and sherry over and stir well. Stand for 30 minutes.
2. Preheat oven to 180°C. Run a sharp knife lightly around the waist of the apple, then place into a baking dish. Stuff the centres of apples with the sultana/date mixture and pour any juice from the glass dish over the apples.
3. Pour remaining pear juice into the baking dish. Bake, covered, for 30–40 minutes, basting with juices from time to time, until apples are tender. Serve with vanilla custard.

Serves 4

VANILLA CUSTARD

1 1/2 tablespoons custard powder
2 cups low-fat milk
1 teaspoon vanilla essence
sugar to taste

1. Blend custard powder and a little milk to a smooth paste.
2. Bring remaining milk to just below boiling point. Whisk in the custard powder paste and simmer, stirring constantly, until custard boils and thickens.
3. Remove from heat and stir in the vanilla essence and sugar to taste.

Makes 2 cups

PEACHES IN RED WINE

4 large peaches
2 cups red wine
1/4 cup caster sugar
1/2 cinnamon stick
2 cloves
grated rind 1 lemon

1. Place peaches into a large bowl. Pour boiling water over

to cover. Let stand for 1 minute, then drain and peel. Cut in half and remove stones.

2. Combine remaining ingredients in a small saucepan. Bring to the boil. Add peaches, reduce heat and simmer for 2–3 minutes. Remove from heat.

3. Spoon peaches and red wine mixture into a bowl. Cover and refrigerate overnight. Serve with sweetened low-fat yoghurt.

Serves 4

11

What partners, family and friends should know

When arthritis strikes it affects not only the patient but also their partner, children, parents, other family members and also close friends. If you're in this position you may not fully understand the implications of this disease; you may want to help but not know what to do; you may also feel a range of conflicting emotions which you don't understand or find hard to deal with. So if your loved one has arthritis, this chapter is for you. For ease of writing I have addressed the text to someone whose partner has arthritis, but the information relates equally well to a child, parent or friend of an arthritis sufferer.

Your first emotion on learning that someone you love has arthritis may be relief to know exactly what is wrong with them, then shock as the implications of the disease sink in, and questions arise.

- Isn't it an old person's disease?
- Will it last long?
- Will she be disabled?
- How is this going to change your life?
- How is it treated?
- Will it affect the family income?
- What medical bills will there be?

You may want to do all you can to help and feel frustrated that you can't do more; or you may find yourself adopting a protective detachment, telling yourself that medical science will find a cure. If your partner doesn't have the energy they once had, is unable to participate in shared activities, needs more help in their daily lives, and can no longer work so your income is affected, you may even feel you've lost your partner in some way. There may be a whole range of changes brought about by the disease which you may be at a loss to deal with, but as these questions, worries and fears are probably the same ones your partner is facing, it's important to share your concerns so that you can find answers together.

Learning about the disease along with your partner can help allay fears for both of you. It will give you the chance to discuss anything that concerns you or anything you don't quite understand, while fostering mutual support which will be strengthening for both of you. You can also become an active member of the 'management team', along with the doctor, specialist, therapists, etc., to support your partner in their efforts to minimise symptoms and maximise quality of life.

Just as an athlete needs a coach to achieve the goal of an Olympic medal, so too do arthritis patients if they are to achieve their goal of well-being. You can be your partner's 'coach'—encouraging them, listening to their concerns, leaving them alone when that's what they want, helping them focus on their goals, cheering them up when they get depressed and generally letting them know that they are not alone in their struggle against the disease. This doesn't mean wrapping them up in cotton wool nor subjugating your life to theirs, but it does mean being practical, and using understanding and consideration towards your partner and all those around you.

No matter what type of arthritis your partner has, the symptoms will normally include stiffness, pain and fatigue. As the severity of symptoms varies from person to person, don't judge your partner by someone else whom you know to have the disease. In some people only one or two joints

111

are affected, symptoms are mild and the impact of the disease is marginal. In others, their whole system may be affected to the point where on bad days they simply can't get out of bed. Remember, your partner is living with a chronic illness; their symptoms may not only vary from day to day, but also from morning to night and the unpredictable nature of arthritis may be hard for them to deal with.

Patients with some forms of the disease, such as rheumatoid arthritis, do go into remission from time to time—periods when the disease becomes less active, symptoms subside and they feel quite well. This remission can last for weeks, months or even years in some cases. However, patients can also experience sudden 'flare-ups' and one of the most frequent comments from people suffering from rheumatoid arthritis is that they can go to bed feeling perfectly well and wake the next morning feeling so ill that it wipes out their day. If your partner experiences a flare-up, rest is important but doesn't necessarily mean bed rest; it can mean taking things easy, wearing a splint or avoiding tasks which would stress their joints.

In general, arthritic pain and stiffness is usually worse in the morning, so your partner may need to have a hot shower and do a few gentle stretching exercises before they can get going. If you live in a household where you have children to get off to school—a hectic time in any household—understanding that your partner may be at their worst at this time of day can help prevent a build-up of tension, resentment on all sides and stormy arguments. A little organisation, such as the children making their own school lunches, or ironing their uniforms the night before, could remove much of the pressure.

UNDERSTANDING WHAT YOUR PARTNER MAY BE FEELING

People have different reactions to being diagnosed with arthritis. Your partner may be feeling one or all of these emotions:

- shock
- denial
- fear
- frustration
- self-pity
- grief
- depression.

These are natural reactions to being faced with chronic illness and coping with symptoms of disease. You can go a long way in helping them—to accept they have the disease, see it as a challenge, and adopt a suitable management plan—by accepting the situation yourself and working with them to lessen the impact of the disease on both your lives.

SHARE THE CHALLENGE

Try imagining that it's you who has the disease—it may help you understand just what your partner is going through. Daily activities, which were once so simple they were hardly a conscious effort, may now be difficult. For a woman, doing up a bra or blow-drying her hair may become a painful experience; for a man simply buttoning his shirt or tying his tie may be a problem. This can be extremely upsetting for the person concerned as it may make them feel helpless and frightened of future incapacity.

By being tuned into your partner's needs you can help them find a different way of doing things. For instance, front fastening bras are common and fashionable and may solve the problem, and some men have found that an old-fashioned button hook makes doing up a shirt easy. Looking for practical, innovative solutions to everyday problems can actually be fun, inspiring and stimulating—it just depends on your attitude.

Your partner will have been prescribed a course of treatment and a management plan. Treatment usually involves taking medication, having physiotherapy and perhaps undergoing surgery. A management plan includes taking medication in strict accordance to the prescription, protecting joints against further damage, rest, exercise, stress and pain control, eating well and losing extra weight if necessary. If possible, accompany your partner to their medical appointments so that you can learn first hand what the situation is, what treatment is recommended and how you can help.

Don't be afraid to ask questions; find out what is happening to your partner's health, why and what the implications are. For example, if it is recommended that your partner no longer carries heavy shopping or mows the lawn, ask why and what will happen if they do. Then you can work out ways around this by having the shopping home delivered or employing someone to cut the grass if you don't have time to do it yourself.

Sometimes when arthritis goes into remission, people can feel so well that they joyfully resume their former lifestyle. They may not take their medication as they should, or protect their joints, or have enough rest. This is an understandable but short-sighted reaction as it may cause more damage to their joints, shortening the period of remission. Help by encouraging them to maintain their management plan, take their medication, exercise and rest when necessary and keep their doctor's appointments.

WHEN A 'FLARE-UP' STRIKES

Flare-ups can strike without warning. One of the most depressing aspects of a disease like rheumatoid arthritis is its unpredictability. Flare-ups may come out of the blue— after a busy period at home or work; just before you go on holiday; or when there is a special family event—without any indications that one is about to occur. They don't seem to be related to any particular pattern of events and no-one knows what triggers them. A severe, unexpected flare-up can be frustrating for everyone, especially if it interferes with some planned activity such as a holiday, or a big social or business occasion. You may feel very frustrated at this time. You may even feel resentment and, at the back of your mind, may even wonder if your partner is malingering. It's important to realise that flare-ups are just as frustrating for your partner as they are for you—and they have to suffer the pain and depression that goes with a flare-up as well. Keep in mind that this is a time when your partner needs your support most, both physically and emotionally. It's a time when the whole family should pull together.

Living with flare-ups means accepting every day as it comes. You may have to learn to be more flexible, adopt a more relaxed attitude to housekeeping, simplify meals by using more pre-prepared foods like ready-made kebabs from your butcher, cook-in sauces for casseroles, healthy take-aways, and generally allow your pace of life to slow. Trying to maintain a hectic schedule will only put pressure on all concerned, and create tension and frustration between you. Being realistic about flare-ups and sensitive to your partner's capabilities will lessen this tension.

WHAT YOU MAY BE FEELING

Living with someone who has a chronic illness, such as arthritis, may produce a number of conflicting emotions. At first it's easy to be understanding and sympathetic, but as time goes by and the illness and subsequent problems don't go away, you may become frustrated, fearful for the future, angry that this has happened to your family and resentful of friends and colleagues who don't have to face these difficulties. You may even feel a desire to run away from it all.

It's sad but true that your life has irrevocably changed, just as your partner's has. You may no longer be able to do the things you once did together. You may have enjoyed skiing, sailing or bush walking which your partner can no longer do. You may feel resentful if you give up these activities, or guilty if you continue to enjoy them when your partner can't. You may even question your right to enjoy yourself when your partner is ill. Financial responsibilities may fall more heavily on you if your partner is unable to maintain his or her income; you may also have to take on once-shared tasks such as cleaning, shopping, washing, gardening, household repairs and car maintenance; you may have to accept more responsibility for looking after the children and dealing with their physical and emotional needs.

You may also have worries of your own, such as fear of losing your job, which you feel you can no longer share with your partner because 'they have enough to cope with'. You may feel overwhelmed by the sheer physical effort and emotional turmoil you're living with. Under these circumstances it's easy to become irritable, moody, angry, frustrated and depressed—and you may find it hard to remain as supportive as you once were.

You may also be feeling guilty for having these emotions—but only saints are perfect and we are only human.

DEALING WITH YOUR EMOTIONS

Feelings of grief, anger, fear, sadness, resentment, embarrassment, denial, frustration and depression are all normal reactions in this situation. However, acknowledging that they are common emotions is not enough to neutralise them. It's important that you find ways of expressing your feelings or they may grow to destroy your relationship.

Here are some effective strategies for dealing with pent up, negative emotions:

- Go somewhere private and have a good cry (even men).
- Discuss the way you feel openly with your partner.
- Express your feelings to someone else you trust.
- Consult your doctor or a family counsellor.
- Approach the Arthritis Foundation, which may be able to refer you to a support group.

It's now recognised that partners of people with chronic illness need help and support too, and talking through your feelings with someone else may help put them into perspective.

TALKING WITH YOUR PARTNER

Even though you might not want to 'burden' your partner with your problems, it's important to talk to them about your feelings. Use the 'I' word instead of 'you' to express the way you feel, then *listen* to what your partner has to say. It can give both of you an insight into each other's lives and problems, bring you closer together and give you a sense of intimacy which is very strengthening.

If you find it difficult to negotiate the minefield of conflicting thoughts and emotions, or have other practical problems, then contact the Arthritis Foundation. It runs education programs and sponsors support groups which you may find helpful at these times.

FIVE STEPS TO STAYING SANE

1. Maintain a sense of humour

Laughter is good medicine for everyone, so even though it is sometimes difficult, try to see the funny side of life. Watch comedy films and videos, go to see your favourite comedian, watch good comedy shows on television. Read humorous novels and listen to humorous audio books on your car radio. Surrounding yourself with wit, comedy and humour can go a long way to lightening the load of living with arthritis.

2. Look on the bright side of life

Positive thinking is a powerful tool in life. Taking an optimistic view and appreciating the good things in your lives can have physical and mental benefits for the whole family. If you believe that there is no problem you can't handle, then there will be none. Focus on what you and your partner can do, not what you can no longer do, live for today and let tomorrow take care of itself.

3. Relax!

Taking active steps to include relaxation in your daily life can be emotionally strengthening, as well as reduce stress and tension. This could mean taking up Tai Chi, yoga, stretch classes or some activity which helps you still your mind, relax your muscles and remove tension from your body. Some people find this in surfing, wood work or lap swimming, while others find it in prayer, visualisation or meditation. Find something that works for you, that you enjoy, look forward to and will practise every day.

4. Keep arthritis in perspective

Don't allow arthritis to become the focus of everyone's lives. Look for the positive in all things. For example, if your partner can no longer kick a football around with the kids, look for another activity you can all do together, such as aqua-volley ball which can be just as much fun with far less wear and tear on the joints. Encourage your partner to take up new interests, and join in them too. Maybe you could learn a foreign language together, take up bridge, or join an amateur dramatic or film society.

5. Make a healthy lifestyle a family thing

Often what is good for an arthritis patient is actually good for everyone. Daily exercise, a well-balanced diet, maintaining normal weight, taking appropriate rest, practising good posture and joint movements, taking an active interest in life, are activities which keep us all fit and healthy.

12

Helping your child overcome arthritis

About one child in every 1000 suffers from some form of juvenile arthritis—a disease rate common throughout the world. Occurring more commonly in girls than boys, it can strike at any age during childhood but appears most often in two age ranges—from one to four years, and during puberty. Most of these children will suffer what is called **acute reactive arthritis** following a bacterial or viral infection, which can be quite severe for a short time but usually disappears in a few weeks or months. However, one in 10,000 children will suffer a more serious form of the disease, which can be much harder to deal with for all concerned.

Coping with childhood illnesses such as chicken pox and mumps is stressful enough, but if your child is diagnosed with a debilitating illness like arthritis it can be particularly difficult. As parents we have an instinctive need to help and protect our children, to take their pain away, to comfort them and make them feel better when they're unwell, but this is often hard when a child has arthritis because of its duration and the physical limitations it places on a child. You may also find it hard to explain why this is happening to them and not to their siblings and friends; how do you help them cope with their pain, discomfort, fatigue and depression; how do you stop yourself worrying about their future; how do you lessen the impact of the disease on the rest of the family?

The good news is that today there is much that can be done to help the child, the parents, siblings and other family members through this experience, so that it has minimal impact on the physical, emotional and social well-being of all concerned.

- *Medically* the outlook is extremely good. Modern drug therapy can now reduce symptoms and relieve pain to the extent that no child needs to suffer unnecessarily.
- *Physically* greater understanding of how arthritis affects joints, muscles and ligaments means these structures can now be protected and strengthened, so the child grows up with little or no damage to their musculo-skeletal system.
- *Educationally* there are many organisations (such as the Arthritis Foundation) and groups you can turn to for help, information and support—parents often feel isolated from close family and friends who are not living with a chronically ill child, and it's comforting to be with people facing similar problems.

Having said this, however, there are three important keys to success:

- First, there must be proper recognition and diagnosis of the disease.
- Second, the child must be treated by appropriate medical specialists, supported by physical and occupational therapists.
- Third, the parents, child, family, relatives, school and friends must be properly informed about all aspects of the disease and ways to deal with it on a day-to-day basis.

FORMS OF JUVENILE ARTHRITIS

The main forms of juvenile arthritis include **systemic onset juvenile arthritis**, **polyarthritis**, **pauciarticular arthritis**,

juvenile ankylosing spondylitis and **adult-type rheumatoid arthritis**.

Systemic onset juvenile arthritis

Affecting both sexes equally, this is usually seen in very young children. The first signs of this disease are fever (which is more intense at night), followed by a rash, enlarged lymph nodes, abdominal pain and weight loss. These symptoms can last for quite a while, in some cases several weeks. Some children experience pain in one or more joints from the onset of the illness, while in others it may take several months for the joints to become swollen, stiff and painful.

Polyarthritis

This can occur in children from infancy onwards and usually affects slightly more girls than boys. Onset of polyarthritis may be sudden, with several joints becoming painful in the course of a few days. In other children, the pain may start in a single joint, then move progressively through others. With this disease, the child may not appear unwell at first other than having painful joints. As the disease progresses however, the child may become tired, listless and reluctant to use the affected limb, holding it in a constant position of least pain. Unfortunately this can lead to stiffness in the joint, and the child should be encouraged to maintain correct posture and limb movement as much as possible.

Pauciarticular arthritis

This is usually seen in toddlers of about two or three years of age, and can go undetected because often the child seems well in themselves. At this age, too, children fall a lot, so a painful joint can be put down to spills rather than arthritis. With this form of arthritis, fewer than four joints are affected and often only a knee joint (**monarticular arthritis**). About one-third of children with pauciarthritis are at risk from eye disease (**chronic iridocyclitis**), which is hard to detect as the eyes don't appear red or painful. It is essential that the

121

child has regular checks-ups by an eye specialist because if left untreated this could eventually lead to blindness.

Juvenile ankylosing spondylitis

This affects more boys than girls, occurring from about the age of ten onwards. It usually involves one or two joints, mainly in the hips and lower back but sometimes also the knees and ankles. As these children may suffer from lower back trouble later in life, caused by inflammation of the joints in the hip girdle, it's vital that they get appropriate medical and physical therapy during their growing years. Children with this form of arthritis are also at risk of eye disease, but it takes a different form to that of pauciarticular arthritis, as the eyes become noticeably red and painful (**acute iridocyclitis**). This condition should be carefully monitored and treated by an ophthalmologist.

Adult-type rheumatoid arthritis

Affecting mainly girls around puberty, this disease attacks the small joints of the hands and feet, but can also cause painful knees and elbows. It is important that it is identified early (there is a blood test which can identify a genetic marker for it), because if left untreated it can cause serious damage to the affected joints.

CAUSES

As with most forms of this disease there is no known cause of juvenile arthritis. What is certain, however, is that it is not caused by going to bed with wet hair, getting soaked by the rain, catching a cold or any of the other old wives' tales that have been attributed to it in the past.

DIAGNOSIS

As the symptoms of juvenile arthritis resemble other childhood illnesses they should be thoroughly investigated to rule out conditions such as viral or bacterial infections, haemophilia or leukaemia. Blood tests may help identify the disease, but arthritis will not be confirmed unless the symptoms persist for more than three months.

TREATMENT

The main aim of treatment is to keep the child's joints as mobile as possible, their muscles strong and their posture correct through their growing years, so that they can reach adulthood with minimal damage to their musculo-skeletal system. Treatment is similar to that for the adult form of the disease in that pain and stiffness in the joints may be relieved by non-steroidal anti-inflammatory drugs and the disease controlled by slow-acting, anti-rheumatic drugs such as gold, penicillamine, sulphasalazine, hydroxychloroquine, metho-trexate and corticosteroids (see 'A–Z guide' for more information on these particular medications).

Many of these drugs are slow acting and may take several weeks or months to show results. It's important that you are encouraging and patient with the child during this period and never change the dose or stop your child's medication without discussing it with their doctor first. If your child reacts badly to any medication, let their doctor know immediately. Different medications suit different children and it may take one or two goes before a suitable one is found.

PHYSICAL THERAPY

Good physical therapy is most important for a child with arthritis to maintain mobility in their joints, increase their muscle tone and keep their ligaments and tendons flexible. Find a physiotherapist you can work well with, because you'll have to help your child with daily movements and exercise, and learn what they should or shouldn't do as far as sport and play is concerned. If a joint is acutely inflamed your child may also have to wear a splint, which most children don't like doing. You must encourage them to be good about this (maybe make some sort of game out of it), as it will reduce the risk of deformity.

Possible side effects from medications for juvenile arthritis

NSAIDs	stomach pain, nausea and vomiting anaemia headache blood in the urine severe abdominal pain and peptic ulcers fragility and scarring of the skin difficulty in concentrating in school, in some cases
Methotrexate	Few side effects have been reported at the dosages at which this drug is usually prescribed. However, your child should be regularly monitored by their doctor as possible side effects could include: diarrhoea low white blood cell count irritation of the lungs mouth sores nausea sinus infection irritation of the liver
Gold	skin rash mouth sores kidney problems low blood count anaemia
Hydroxychloroquine (Plaquenil)	upset stomach skin rash damage to the eyes. A child taking this drug should be checked every six to twelve months by an ophthalmologist.

(*Note*: It's important that this drug is kept well out of reach of small children as an overdose can be fatal.)

Corticosteroids	If taken over a long period of time these may: increase blood pressure cause osteoporosis (softening of the bones) slow the child's growth rate reduce resistance to infection produce sudden mood swings increase appetite lead to weight gain increase the risk for ulcers

While on any medication, if your child displays any of the symptoms mentioned above, consult their doctor immediately.

EXERCISE FOR CHILDREN WITH ARTHRITIS

Exercise is vitally important for children with juvenile arthritis, to lessen the effects of the disease on their growing bodies. Exercise includes:

- therapeutic exercises which help the child walk, sit, stand

and perform functions such as writing, in a way least likely to damage their joints

- range-of-motion exercises which will keep their joints flexible. If performed after a warm bath or shower these can ease morning stiffness and help to maintain flexibility and strength (ask your physiotherapist about these exercises and see Chapter 9).
- strengthening exercises to build or maintain muscles and muscle tone
- recreational activities, such as swimming, to mobilise joints, muscles and ligaments and help keep your child supple while maintaining strength and fitness.

If your child wants to play sport then it's doubly important that they build strong muscles and learn to protect their joints properly. Discuss this with their doctor as some sports may not be appropriate while others may need some special training or protective equipment in order for the child to participate.

WHAT ELSE MAY HELP?

Just as with adult arthritis, pain and stiffness can be eased with heat, so warm baths and showers may be very comforting to a child, as will heat packs and hot water bottles. Distraction also works well with children so if they are feeling miserable and out of sorts, tell them a story, let them watch a funny video or play a new computer game—it can really take them out of themselves.

FEEDING YOUR CHILD WELL

Even the healthiest child can be picky over food, but a child with arthritis can be even more choosy about what they eat. This can prove a real headache for parents anxious to ensure their child is receiving adequate nourishment.

When children are sick they usually only want familiar, comforting food—it makes them feel safe and secure. It can be very reassuring for them to eat the same food day after day, so don't worry if they choose to eat a limited range, or want just one type of food—such as peanut butter sandwiches or macaroni cheese—for every meal. It's best not to make an issue out of it. Just go along with what the child wants but have snacks on hand such as fruit and vegetables (sliced apples or bananas, vegetable match sticks, fruit smoothies, etc.), so the child can help themselves without being asked. Even if they only nibble on these they'll be consuming important nutrients.

Try these strategies:

- If they won't drink milk, try tempting them with flavoured milk-shakes, frozen yoghurt, ice-cream, cheese sticks, custards and other milk puddings.
- If they leave their vegetables on the side of the plate, offer them vegetable sticks with a bowl of cottage cheese to dip into as a snack. Or puree the vegetable and serve it as a soup, or juice a selection and see if they will take it as a drink.
- Fruit can be cooked, pureed and served in desserts, blended into smoothies, or sliced into thin wedges and served with a fruit yoghurt for dipping.
- If they're reluctant to eat meat, try offering it to them as finger food—most children love eating with their hands. Hamburgers are popular with most children, as are chicken legs, lamb cutlets, etc. If they can pick food up with their hands they will usually eat at least some of it. If they still won't eat meat, then give them protein in the form of eggs, peanut butter, baked beans or lentils.

A FAMILY AFFAIR

One of the most important challenges for parents is to help their arthritic child and the rest of the family adapt as well as possible to the situation and not let it take all the joy and wonder out of life. Here are some strategies to try:

- Try to give equal time to all children in the family. Sometimes parents can become so focused on a sick child that the siblings feel neglected and then become

AVERAGE NUTRITIONAL DAILY REQUIREMENTS FOR A CHILD

Bread and cereals (provide energy, B group vitamins, iron and fibre)—5–6 servings

One serving = 1 slice bread
2 breakfast cereal biscuits
1/2 cup cooked pasta, rice or noodles
2 large wholemeal biscuits or crackers

Fruit and vegetables (provide vitamins A and C, folic acid, energy and fibre)—4 servings

One serving = 1 piece fruit
3–4 pieces dried fruit
1/2 cup fruit salad
1/2 cup fruit or vegetable juice
1/4 cup cooked vegetables
1 small potato
1/2 raw carrot or celery stick

Milk and dairy products (provide calcium, protein, riboflavin, vitamins A and D)—3 servings (600 mL total)

One serving = 200 mL milk
200 g tub yoghurt
1 cup milk custard
30 g slice cheese

Meat, eggs, pulses (provide protein, iron, B group vitamins and zinc)—2 servings

One serving = 30 g cooked meat, chicken or fish
1 egg
1/2 cup cooked beans, lentils or pulses
1 tablespoon peanut butter

Fats (provide vitamins A, D and E and essential fatty acids)—no more than 20 g (4 teaspoons) butter, margarine or oil resentful and jealous. By explaining the disease to all your children and giving each of them special time and attention, it can turn siblings into helpful allies rather than disruptive monsters. Sick children can often get great strength and comfort from supportive brothers and sisters, who in turn can learn some valuable lessons about compassion and understanding from the experience.

- Try to maintain as normal a household as possible. Don't wrap your sick child up in cotton wool. Allowing them to rest on the couch watching television while their brothers and sisters have to wash up or tidy their rooms isn't going to lead to household harmony; it could also have a negative impact on the child's character by encouraging the belief that they should always be waited on. Work out chores that the child *can* do (warm washing up water can be quite soothing for sore fingers) and don't let the illness become an excuse for laziness. By maintaining your normal expectations of behaviour and activities you'll help downplay the impact the disease is having on all family members.

- Help your children understand what arthritis is all about. Give them material, appropriate for their age, which explains what is involved and how the disease is treated, then go through it with them and let them have their own copy to read or look at by themselves. Encourage them to ask questions and address their worries and fears.

- Talk to your child's school about the situation. Sometimes children with arthritis experience difficulties because their teachers and schoolmates don't understand their condition, have no idea about the nature of the illness or know what to expect from a child with arthritis.

- Try to encourage relatives—especially grandparents—to treat the child in the same way they always have and not make more of a fuss over them than over your other children.

- Remember to allow some time for yourselves, individually and together. Parents can be consumed by the emotional and physical load of dealing with work, home, family and a sick child, at a cost to themselves and their relationship. So make sure you have time to relax and spend time together as people rather than just parents. It will give you the strength to carry on.

If at any time you feel that you can't cope, then contact the Arthritis Foundation which has skilled counsellors willing and able to listen to your concerns, provide helpful advice and information and which can also refer you on to other support groups and agencies. Despite the challenges this disease will present to you and your family, you can achieve the goal of helping your child and other family members to enjoy life. This means minimising the impact arthritis has on the family and maximising the fun and laughter that comes with family life.

Part 2

Understanding arthritis

An A–Z guide
to arthritis

INTRODUCTION

In this A–Z guide you'll find descriptions of the main forms of arthritis, including their symptoms, diagnosis and treatment. It also includes the types of drugs used in treatment and possible side effects you may experience. I have also included alternative therapies reputed to give some relief from symptoms which may complement your medical treatment. While I believe that modern pharmaceuticals, physical therapies and surgical procedures are extremely effective in the treatment of arthritis, I don't have a closed mind to complementary therapies which may also have a role to play in managing symptoms. I would not for a moment suggest you replace conventional medicine with alternative therapies, but I feel that if you find them helpful in reducing pain, managing stress, or lifting depression, then there is no harm in *adding* them to your treatment program, so long as you tell your doctor about what you are doing.

ACUPRESSURE

This is an ancient Chinese healing technique, which uses pressure points on the body to stimulate the flow of energy and improve circulation. Instead of using needles, acupressure uses the thumbs, palms, heels of the hands and elbows (sometimes also knees and feet) to stimulate vital points around the body. Along with this pressure point treatment, gentle stretching and corrective exercises are also used. Less invasive than acupuncture, this therapy is said to be helpful in relieving the pain and stiffness of arthritis.

ACUPUNCTURE

Acupuncture is another ancient Chinese healing technique which uses fine needles to activate healing points throughout the body. It's based on the belief that our life force, known as chi, flows through our bodies along twelve paths or meridians. Illness is thought to occur when the flow of chi becomes blocked, or stagnant, upsetting the body's balance and function. Very fine needles are inserted into specific points along these energy meridians to restore the healing flow of chi throughout the body. In arthritis, these needles are used to stimulate the release of endorphins in the brain, helping to close the 'pain gate', to promote better circulation and open up blocked meridians. Some arthritis sufferers have found that acupuncture does relieve chronic pain.

ALEXANDER TECHNIQUE

Developed by Frederick Mathias Alexander, this therapy focuses on improving the body's natural posture, balance and movement and thereby increasing overall physical and psychological well-being. Alexander believed that many of us exist in a state of physical tension, especially if we are suffering from chronic illnesses such as arthritis. This tension causes poor posture, encourages the body to sag, the spine to distort and muscles to shorten, causing stiffness, backache, fatigue and depression. Alexander believed we could reverse this by careful self-observation, and learning to release these tensions through movement and correct posture.

An Alexander teacher uses verbal and gentle hands-on instructions to reveal the tension in your body and teach you ways to release it. By learning to tune into your body you will find it easier to recognise when you are becoming tense and develop the ability to relax both your mind and body at will, which can be helpful in overcoming pain, muscle tension and improving your overall flexibility.

ALLOPURINAL

This is a drug used to prevent recurrent attacks of gout. It's an enzyme inhibitor which helps prevent the formation of uric acid crystals. In a few people it can produce some side effects such as a skin rash, fever, headache and stomach upset. When on this medication it is important to avoid alcohol, which could negate its effectiveness. You should also let your doctor or chemist know you are taking it when being prescribed other medication, as some drugs can interfere with its action.

ANALGESICS

Analgesics are used to relieve arthritis pain caused in conditions where there is little inflammation, such as osteoarthritis and soft-tissue rheumatism. These pain killers include paracetamol and codeine. Side effects may include:

- *paracetamol*—adverse side effects are rare, however, it may cause nausea or a rash in isolated cases
- *codeine*—may cause dizziness or drowsiness, especially if alcohol is consumed at the same time; if taken over a long time it may cause constipation and dependency.

ANGELICA

Both Western and Oriental herbalists claim that this herb has anti-inflammatory properties which can help relieve the pain and stiffness of arthritis. It can be made into a tea and taken twice a day, or taken in tincture form as 1 teaspoon twice a day. It should not be given to children under 2 years of age, and children and people over 65 should only take low-strength doses.

Caution: Taking angelica can cause a skin rash if you go out into the sun.

ANKYLOSING SPONDYLITIS

A disease which affects almost one in 100 people, ankylosing spondylitis is inflammation of the joints in the spine, which causes stiffness and rigidity. It affects more men than women, often when they are in their twenties and thirties. There appears to be an hereditary factor associated with this disease—if you have a close relative with the disease then your chances of developing it are increased. If left untreated, this condition can lead to permanent stiffness of the spine, restricted mobility and freedom of movement.

Symptoms

Stiffness, especially in the morning, in the hips and lower back, is usually the first noticeable symptom. Back pain may develop and mobility decrease as the disease progresses. Some patients may also suffer pain in other joints such as their knees, heels, ankles and chest where the ribs join the spine. Fatigue, listlessness, lack of appetite and, occasionally, painful eyes due to inflammation of the iris (iritis) may also be experienced.

Diagnosis

This is usually made from reported symptoms, blood tests to identify a genetic marker called HLA-B27, and spinal x-rays to determine the condition of the vertebrae.

Treatment

There is no cure for this disease so treatment relies on managing the condition. Anti-inflammatory drugs as well as physical therapies, such as heat treatment, massage, gentle exercise and mobilisation by a physiotherapist, are all employed in the management of the disease. Daily gentle exercise such as swimming is essential to maintain strength in the back muscles. Developing correct posture is vital and learning strategies like the Alexander Technique can help prevent curvature of the spine. See also **backache**.

ANTI-INFLAMMATORIES

These are medications designed to reduce the symptoms of inflammation, i.e. pain, swelling, redness and heat. These include non-steroidal anti-inflammatories (NSAIDs) and corticosteroid drugs.

Foods which are said to have anti-inflammatory properties include: apples, blackcurrants, fish oil (omega-3 fatty acids), garlic, ginger, hot chilli peppers, onion, pineapple and sage.

AROMATHERAPY

Aromatherapy is the use of pure essential oils from aromatic plants. From the ancient civilisations of China, India and Egypt onwards, healers have used aromatic oils to speed recovery of wounds, ward off disease, alter moods and relieve common ailments.

Interest in these oils in the West was rekindled after World War I when a French doctor discovered that lavender oil was effective in healing the wounds of soldiers burned and injured during the war. Intrigued by this discovery, he went on to investigate the healing properties of other plant oils. His work inspired other researchers and spawned modern aromatherapy practice, so that today many people are recognising the power and effectiveness of this ancient healing art.

Aromatherapy is based on the idea that our sense of smell is closely linked to our memory and emotions. It's this response which is used in aromatherapy to influence our moods, relax our muscles and create a sense of well-being.

Essential oils can be added to baths, blended into massage oils, used as a compress or inhalation, and also in special burners which fill the room with fragrance; they can be used to relieve stress and tension, soothe aches and pains, and lift your mood.

(**Caution**: Essential oil should never be taken internally.)

Only a few drops of oil are required for any of these uses and combinations of oil can improve their effectiveness.

Use for a massage oil added to 50 mL of almond oil

- To relieve the symptoms of rheumatism—10 drops juniper oil, 10 drops lemon oil and 5 drops thyme oil.
- To relax muscle tension before sleep—8 drops sage oil, 8 drops cypress oil, 6 drops benzoin oil and 6 drops chamomile oil.
- For general use in rheumatism—8 drops rosemary oil, 8 drops juniper oil, 6 drops thyme oil and 6 drops eucalyptus oil; or 9 drops lavender oil, 8 drops cypress oil and 6 drops ginger oil.
- For rheumatic flare-up—9 drops pine oil, 9 drops rosemary oil and 9 drops ginger oil.

Use in a burner

Half-fill the top dish with water and add the essential oils to it. Light the night light candle below, and as the water warms the essential oil will vaporise, releasing its aroma.

- To lift depression—2 drops geranium oil, 2 drops clary sage oil and 2 drops bergamot oil.
- To ease anxiety—3 drops lavender oil, 2 drops bergamot oil and 1 drop patchouli oil.
- To lift fatigue and boost energy—2 drops rosemary oil, 2 drops basil oil and 2 drops lemon oil.

Use in a bath

- To ease general aches and pains—5 drops angelica oil.
- To relieve tension—3 drops bergamot oil, 2 drops lavender oil and 1 drop cedarwood oil.

Note: Essential oils, like all medicines, should be stored well out of the reach of children.

ARTHRODESIS

This is an operation in which the bones in a joint are fused in order to relieve pain, correct deformity or prevent instability. Once fused the joint is permanently rigid, but it will be stronger, more stable and no longer painful. It's usually recommended where all other treatments such as medication, physiotherapy or splinting have failed and reconstruction isn't an option. If performed on larger joints, such as in the spine, it is done under a general anaesthetic, but smaller joints, such as in the fingers, can be fused under local anaesthetic.

Procedures vary depending on the joint concerned but, in general, the cartilage from the ends of the bones is removed, then the surface layer of bone shaved away. The ends of the bones are drawn together and held in place by screws, plates or rods while new bone cells grow and fuse the two bones together.

ARTHROPLASTY

This term describes a range of joint reconstruction procedures. Although knee or hip replacements are the most common operations, it can also be performed on the elbows, fingers, shoulders, jaw and ankles (see 'Surgery', page 164, for more detail).

ARTHROSCOPY

One of the most common orthopaedic procedures performed today, arthroscopy is usually recommended for people suffering from osteoarthritis when joint damage is first suspected. It allows the surgeon to inspect the inside of a joint, such as the knee, to assess how much damage has been done by the disease, as this does not always show up on x-rays. During the procedure the surgeon can also remove loose material or fluid from the joint for further examination, repair torn cartilage and ligaments, or shave and smooth the surface of the kneecap.

Two small incisions are made either side of the knee and an endoscope (a fine optical tube attached to a television monitor) is inserted into the joint. The endoscope allows the surgeon to examine the condition of the bones, cartilage and synovium and carry out remedial work. The procedure is usually performed under general anaesthetic but can be carried out as day surgery. However, the patient may be kept in overnight if the operation takes place in the late afternoon.

AUTOIMMUNE DISEASE

Autoimmune disease, which includes rheumatoid arthritis and systemic lupus erythematosus (SLE), occurs when the body's defence and repair mechanisms go wrong. A normal immune system is composed of cells and their products including antibodies. These antibodies are proteins designed to fight off invading bacteria and viruses, to protect against tissue damage and to promote healing. In autoimmune diseases these antibodies and cells start to attack and injure healthy body tissue. Medical science has yet to find the cause of this malfunction and treatment of these diseases is similar to rheumatoid arthritis (see page 160 for more details).

AZATHIOPRINE

This is an immunosuppressant drug used in the treatment of severe, active rheumatoid arthritis, which has not responded to other 'first-line' medications. It can have side effects which include nausea, vomiting, loss of appetite, a reduced sperm count in men, and a lowering of the white blood cell count. All patients on this medication should have regular blood counts and liver function tests.

BACKACHE

Backache is a common symptom of some forms of arthritis such as osteoarthritis and ankylosing spondylitis. To help prevent back pain it's important to stay physically fit, avoid becoming overweight, maintain good posture and adopt good carrying and lifting techniques. Here are four ways to reduce backache:

1. When sitting, at a desk or in a lounge chair, make sure you keep your upper back straight and your shoulders relaxed. Try not to slump in the chair with your bottom towards the front and your lower back curved and unsupported. Keep your stomach muscles tight and maintain the natural arch in your lower back by supporting it with a back support or cushion.
2. Do daily exercises to strengthen your stomach muscles, which do most of the work in supporting your back. Lie on the floor with your knees bent, hands crossed on your chest. Curl your head and shoulders off the floor as if you were trying to look at your toes. Hold for a count of 5, then return to starting position. Start off with 4–5 repeats and gradually work up to 20 or more.
3. If you are carrying any extra weight on your tummy then make an effort to lose it because it can strain your lower back and weaken your stomach muscles.
4. Two stretches to relieve an aching back:
   a) Lie on your back and raise your knees to your chest. Clasp them with your arms and rest in this position for 2–3 minutes, then slowly lower your legs.
   b) Lie on your stomach, with legs straight and arms under your shoulders. Now push yourself up onto your elbows into the sphinx position. Don't strain, just relax and let your hips sink onto the floor. Hold for 3–4 minutes. You should feel the ache in your back gather towards the centre and then ease. If, however, pain radiates away from your spine or down your leg, stop this stretch immediately and consult your doctor. If any back pain persists for more than a day or two you should consult your doctor about it.

BURSITIS

Bursitis is inflammation of the bursa, a fluid-filled sac that acts as a gliding surface between moving body tissue to stop muscles or tendons rubbing against bone or other muscles, such as in the knee, elbow, shoulder or big toe. Inflammation of the bursa can be caused by rheumatoid arthritis or gout, as well as by injury to the surrounding area.

Rest and the application of cold packs to the affected area will help reduce the pain and swelling and the condition will normally disappear within a few days. If this simple treatment doesn't work, then your doctor may draw off the excess fluid using a syringe, then apply a pressure bandage to stop the bursa filling up again. It may also be recommended that the bursa is injected with a corticosteroid drug to speed recovery.

CARTILAGE

Cartilage is a smooth, tough material covering the ends of bones in joints, which acts as a shock absorber and allows the joint to move easily.

CHAPARRAL

Chaparral or creosote bush is native to Mexico and the south-western states of the USA. Herbalists believe it to have anti-inflammatory and antioxidant properties which may help in the fight against arthritis. A tea can be made from the twigs and bark but it has a most unpleasant taste, so you may have to blend it with other herbal teas and flavour it with honey and lemon to make it acceptable.

CHIROPRACTIC

Chiropractors believe there is a life force within all of us which animates, heals and motivates every cell and molecule in our bodies. This life force is coordinated by the brain and flows around the body through the nervous system. As the spine is the central carrier of the nervous system, faults or defects in its structure can interfere with this flow of healing energy and result in disease in various parts of the body.

Chiropractors seek out these interferences, called subluxations, and manipulate the body to realign the spine and nervous system, thus freeing up the life force to do its healing work. They also work to keep the spine as flexible as possible because they believe the more supple our spines become, the more able we are to recover from illness.

COLCHICINE

Colchicine is a medication used to suppress inflammation in acute attacks of gout, thus reducing the pain and swelling caused by uric acid crystal deposits. It can cause side effects such as weakness, hair loss, nausea, vomiting, abdominal pains and diarrhoea. It may also damage bone marrow so all patients on this medication require careful blood count monitoring.

CORTICOSTEROIDS

For conditions such as osteoarthritis, rheumatoid arthritis, gout, seronegative arthritis, tenosynovitis, bursitis, tendinitis and tennis elbow, an injection of corticosteroid into the joint, or soft tissue surrounding it, brings rapid relief from pain and swelling by reducing inflammation. The benefits are seen within hours and can last for up to six weeks. Although most joints can be injected, it is particularly helpful in the knee and shoulder. As corticosteroid injections are given only occasionally, side effects are rare. However, oral corticosteroids can have substantial side effects and so are only prescribed when other medication has been ineffective. Possible side effects include:

- redistribution of body fat (appearing more around the face and trunk)
- increased appetite
- weight gain
- thinner, more fragile skin

- increased susceptibility to infection
- mood swings
- cataracts
- increased blood pressure
- salt and fluid retention.

DEVIL'S CLAW

This is a South American plant believed to have analgesic and anti-inflammatory properties by the native Indians. Commercially developed in Germany as a herbal remedy, it can be made into a decoction or taken as a tincture three times a day.

DIATHERMY

This is a heat treatment which uses short-wave radio and electromagnetic fields to bring quick pain relief to arthritis sufferers.

DISEASE-MODIFYING ANTI-RHEUMATIC DRUGS (DMARDS)

These medications are used to treat various forms of arthritis including rheumatoid arthritis, systemic lupus erythematosus (SLE), seronegative arthritis, psoriatic arthritis and ankylosing spondylitis. Although it's not known just how they work, and while not a cure, they will relieve symptoms and minimise joint, cartilage and bone damage. Common DMARDs include:

- anti-malarial hydroxychloroquine (Plaquenil)
- sulphasalazine (Salazopyrin EN)
- gold compounds (Auranofin and Myocrisin)
- D-penicillamine (D-Penamine)
- methotrexate (Ledertrexate, Methoblastin).

These are powerful, but slow-acting drugs (except Methotrexate, see page 153) which may take three to four months to show benefits. However, improvements are normally substantial with many patients reporting decreased inflammation, pain relief, greater mobility, and increased energy levels.

A few people do experience some side effects from these drugs, but careful monitoring can pick up any problem quickly and appropriate action then taken. Most patients, however, feel the benefits of taking DMARDs far outweigh any risks of side effects.

D-PENICILLAMINE

This is a disease-modifying drug used to control rheumatoid arthritis by reducing inflammation and preventing flare-ups. It's a drug that works well in some people and not others. The dose is usually started low and increased slowly over a matter of weeks. Possible side effects include skin rashes, sore gums, mouth ulcers, loose bowel motions, reduced white blood cell and platelet counts, change in kidney function, and temporary loss of taste. However, when prescribed in small doses these can be minimised. This medication should not be taken at the same time as iron supplements, antacids or Guinness, as they can reduce its effectiveness. Regular blood and urine tests should be performed to monitor the effects of this treatment.

ENDORPHINS

Morphine-like, pain-killing substances released by the brain.

ESR

This is a test called erythrocyte sedimentation rate and is used to assess the degree of disease activity in rheumatoid arthritis. A high ESR means the disease is very active.

FELDENKRAIS METHOD

According to famous anthropologist Margaret Mead, 'This is the most sophisticated and effective method I have seen for the prevention and reversal of deterioration of function', and world renowned violinist Yehudi Menuhin claimed, 'The Feldenkrais exercises are ingenious and simple'. These are just two of the countless people who claimed to have been helped by this gentle mobilising technique.

It was developed by American physicist Dr Moshe Feldenkrais who, after personal injury, set out to develop a way for people to achieve physical and mental well-being in a gentle and sustaining way. In order to understand how the human body works he studied the movements of children, then developed a set of movements designed to encourage adults to regain the kind of flexibility and ease of movement they had in childhood.

The Feldenkrais Method involves a series of slow, subtle, and sometimes unusual movements. Students are taught to be aware of which muscles they are using in each movement and in repeating an unfamiliar movement many times the brain learns a new range of motion. Dr Feldenkrais has worked with people suffering from arthritis, curvature of the spine, stroke, cerebral palsy and multiple sclerosis.

Each lesson concentrates on a particular movement. There is a slow development of ability through a series of carefully orchestrated manoeuvres which are performed as slowly as possible, without strain; after 15 or 20 repetitions the initial effort drops to practically nothing. It is claimed that training the body this way not only improves its strength and flexibility, but makes a profound change in the health and well-being of the student.

GOLD (AURANOFIN AND MYOCRISIN)

Gold compounds have been used to treat rheumatoid arthritis for a long time, however, patient response can be quite varied. For some people it's the best drug for controlling their disease and they experience long-term remission, while others gain little benefit. Gold therapy comes in two forms: Auranofin (oral gold) and Myocrisin (injectable gold). Unfortunately, about 30 per cent of patients have to stop this treatment because they experience skin rashes, sore gums, mouth ulcers, loose bowel motions, reduced white blood cell and platelet counts, and changes in kidney function. If gold injections are prescribed for you, then you should have your urine and blood checked before each injection.

GOUT

Gout is one of the most common types of arthritis. Affecting ten times as many men as women, there is usually a family history of the disease. Gout in men can occur any time after puberty, though onset is usually between 40 and 50 years of age. Women tend to experience it only after the menopause.

Symptoms

Gout normally affects only one joint, usually the big toe, however, it can occur in the ankle, knee, elbow, wrist or hand. Onset of an attack can be sudden, such as overnight. The joint rapidly becomes swollen, red and painful, with pain increasing over the next day or so. The pain has been described as excruciating to the point where even the touch of a bed sheet is agony.

An initial bout usually only lasts a few days and some people never experience another one. Others, unfortunately, have further attacks, the second coming between six months to two years later. The more attacks of gout you have, the more frequent they may become and the more joints will be involved. Repeated attacks can also accelerate joint damage leading to persistent pain.

Cause

Gout is caused by uric acid crystal deposits in a joint, although they can also be deposited in soft tissue around tendons and in the ears. It's a metabolic disorder and may also be associated with the presence of kidney stones.

Uric acid is normally dissolved in the blood stream and excreted out through the kidneys. However, if the body can't get rid of the uric acid fast enough, it concentrates in the blood (hyperuricaemia). As a result, uric acid crystals precipitate into the joint spaces and surrounding tissue. These crystals irritate the synovium, triggering the inflammatory process which produces the classic symptoms of heat, redness, pain and swelling.

Bouts of gout often occur for no obvious reason but may be triggered by:

- alcohol
- over-eating
- superficial injury to a joint
- dehydration
- crash diets
- fasting.

Diagnosis

This is usually made from symptoms and by a blood test—an excessive level of uric acid would confirm the disease. However, sometimes no elevated levels of uric acid are found and it may be necessary to take fluid from the joint for examination under a microscope. The presence of uric acid crystals would confirm the diagnosis.

Treatment

Today, due to medical advances, gout can be well managed and doesn't have to cause the pain and suffering experienced by previous generations. Being overweight, drinking too much alcohol and not drinking enough fluids can aggravate this condition, so paying attention to these factors can go a long way to preventing further attacks.

The pain and inflammation in the joint can be relieved by taking non-steroidal anti-inflammatory drugs (NSAIDs). Treatment should start as early as possible to minimise damage to the joint, and if you are subject to recurring attacks of gout you should always have your medication handy and commence taking it as soon as possible. As the pain and swelling subsides, usually within a few days, the medication is tapered off and finally stopped once the attack is over. If the inflammation is not responding to the NSAID,

A knee affected by gout

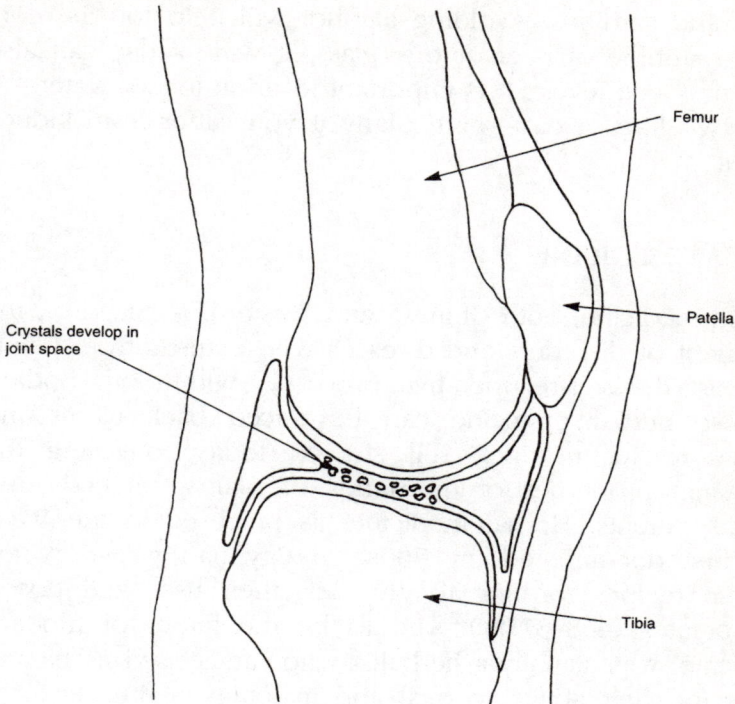

Femur

Patella

Crystals develop in
joint space

Tibia

then colchicine may be prescribed; if that isn't effective a
corticosteroid drug may be injected directly into the joint.

For long-term management of this condition, drugs such
as probenicid or sulfinpyrazone may be prescribed to lower
uric acid levels in the blood and allow it to be passed
through the kidneys and excreted in urine. If uric acid levels
in the blood remain persistently high then you may need to
be on drug therapy for life in order to avoid complications
such as kidney disease and high blood pressure.

Diet can play an important role in the management of
gout. If you are overweight your body may not be as efficient
as it should be in getting rid of uric acid, so shedding those
extra kilos is important, as is watching what you eat and
drink.

Purine can elevate uric acid in the blood so people who
suffer from gout should avoid foods containing it such as

liver, kidney, brains, sweetbreads, anchovies, poultry, pulses, yeast and sardines. Avoiding alcohol will help too as more than a stubbie of beer or one glass of wine a day can also raise uric acid levels. It is important to drink lots of water—at least two litres a day—particularly if you suffer from kidney stones.

HERBAL MEDICINE

Herbal medicine, both Chinese and Western, is based on the treatment of disorders and diseases with extracts from plants to assist the self-recuperative processes within our bodies. Chinese herbal medicine can be traced back to around 2500BC to manuscripts, still studied today, outlining the medicinal properties of thousands of plants, minerals and animal extracts. Herbal medicine, as practised in the West, was first documented in 1700BC in Egyptian papyri which contain recipes for herbal remedies, their uses and doses. Hippocrates (468–377BC), said to be the father of modern medicine, was actually a herbalist who categorised herbs and foods for their ability to heal and maintain health.

Down through the centuries, all doctors and healers have turned to plants for their healing qualities and it wasn't until the late 19th and 20th centuries, with the discovery of antibiotics and the development of modern pharmaceuticals, that traditional herbal medicines lost favour with doctors.

Common herbal remedies for arthritis include angelica, chaparral, Devil's claw, horsetail, juniper, yucca and zingiber (see separate listings).

HORSETAIL

The Chinese have long held the belief that horsetail—a bamboo-like marsh dweller—is a cure for arthritis. It has now been found that horsetail has the ability to absorb gold dissolved in water. As gold is used in the treatment of rheumatoid arthritis there may be some truth to this ancient belief. However, as long-term use of this herb can deplete the body's potassium stores, it's best to discuss it with your doctor or a qualified herbalist before taking it.

HYDROTHERAPY

These are gentle exercises performed in warm water and supervised by a trained instructor. It is designed to maintain mobility, strengthen muscles and increase joint flexibility.

HYDROXYCHLOROQUINE

This is an antimalarial drug used in the treatment of auto-immune diseases such as rheumatoid arthritis and SLE to improve symptoms in patients with early active disease, where only a few joints are affected. There is a slight risk of eye problems with this drug so it's important to have your eyes examined twice yearly and to avoid long exposure to strong sunlight.

INFECTIVE ARTHRITIS

This is caused by bacterial infection of a joint, either directly from the blood stream or through an open wound. The immune system triggers the inflammatory response and the familiar symptoms of warmth, redness, swelling and pain follow. Other viruses and infections, such as chickenpox, German measles, gonorrhoea, mumps and rheumatic fever may also cause arthritis in some joints.

INFLAMMATION

This is the body's normal response to injury or disease. It triggers the release of chemicals which increases blood flow to the area. The increase in blood means greater numbers of white blood cells are available to heal and repair tissue. Symptoms include warmth, swelling, stiffness and pain in the affected area.

JUNIPER

Long thought to have anti-inflammatory properties, studies in Germany (where herbal medicine is used far more widely in mainstream medicine) have shown that drinking juniper tea can relieve the pain and stiffness of rheumatoid arthritis. A tea can be made by infusing 1 teaspoon of lightly crushed berries in 1 cup of boiling water, then steeping for 10 minutes. Herbalists recommend drinking no more than two cups a day for no more than six weeks.

Caution: Juniper can cause kidney irritation and should not be taken by anyone with a kidney problem; it may also cause an allergic reaction in some people. It is best to consult a qualified herbalist before trying this remedy.

KALE

Including generous amounts of kale in your diet is said to be beneficial for those suffering from autoimmune diseases, such as rheumatoid arthritis and SLE. A member of the cabbage family, it is rich in antioxidants and other chemicals which are thought to boost the immune system and protect body tissues from attack. Resembling a curly silverbeet, the thick ribs should be removed and the leaves steamed in just the water clinging to them after washing. It can be used in any dish in a similar way to silverbeet and spinach.

LIQUORICE

Herbalists believe that liquorice has both anti-inflammatory and anti-arthritic properties, and is especially useful in treating rheumatoid arthritis. It can be taken either as a tea or a tincture, however, it is best prescribed by a qualified herbalist or naturopath as taking too much liquorice can raise blood pressure and should not be taken by pregnant women.

LUPUS

See Systemic lupus erythematosus (SLE).

METHOTREXATE

This is an immunosuppressant drug used to treat rheumatoid and psoriatic arthritis. It's a faster acting, disease-modifying anti-rheumatic drug showing benefits in four to six weeks, rather than the three to four months of other types. Initially there were concerns about short- and long-term adverse effects from taking this drug, but it has now been shown that they are minimised when taken strictly in accordance with the prescription and the patient is carefully monitored. Tablets should be taken once a week, with the dose starting low and gradually increasing at monthly intervals. Minor side effects may include nausea, fatigue, abdominal discomfort, sore mouth, reduced white blood cell and platelet count and changes in liver function.

Taking folic acid can help reduce side effects like nausea, fatigue, abdominal discomfort and sore mouth and monthly tests may be required to monitor blood and liver functions. It's important that pregnancy is avoided and alcohol limited.

NATUROPATHY

Naturopathy is based on the belief that the body has the ability to heal itself when free of toxins that have accumulated through unhealthy lifestyle habits. A naturopath will diagnose and treat a patient who is suffering from pain, injury or disease by stimulating the body's natural defences and promoting an equilibrium that allows the body to function properly and effectively. This therapy may involve changes in diet, exercise, massage and other manipulative therapies as well as natural remedies.

NEUROSURGERY

Neurosurgery can sometimes bring relief to those suffering

from severe rheumatoid arthritis where the disease is affecting their hands. Inflammation of the coverings of the tendons or tendon sheaths, known as carpal tunnel compression, can cause numbness, tingling in the fingers and pain in the thumb. If treatments such as splinting or cortisone injections have failed, then neurosurgery may be the only answer.

NON-STEROIDAL ANTI-INFLAMMATORY DRUGS (NSAIDS)

These are some of the most widely prescribed drugs in Australia. NSAIDs reduce inflammation, ease day-to-day joint pain and stiffness and help slow down the progress of the disease. There are a number on the market and different brands suit different people. Trial and error will sort out which one is best for you. If you're prescribed a NSAID it's important to understand the correct dosage, and how it should be taken (i.e. with or after food, at night, or with plenty of fluid).

NSAIDs include:

- non-salicylate NSAIDs (Clinoril, Indocid, Arthrexin)
- oxicam derivatives (Feldene, Tilcotil)
- phenylacetic acid derivatives (Voltaren)
- propionic acid derivatives (Brufen, Nurofen, Orudis, Naprosyn, Surgam).

Relief from symptoms is relatively fast, usually between two to three days, but it could take up to one or two weeks. However, if there is no improvement after that time, see your doctor who may prescribe another NSAID.

NSAIDs usually come as tablets or capsules although there are also rectal suppositories. Some people do experience mild side effects from NSAIDs including:

- stomach upset
- indigestion, heartburn or nausea
- dizziness
- headache
- skin allergies.

If you experience any of these symptoms, tell your doctor immediately. Also tell your doctor if you:

- have a change in bowel habits
- vomit blood or pass bowel motions containing blood which sometimes makes the stool black (stop the NSAID immediately if you notice this)
- are planning a pregnancy, already pregnant or breastfeeding.

OSTEOARTHRITIS

Osteoarthritis is the most common form of arthritis affecting a large proportion of the population over the age of 60, although it can also occur in younger people. It affects women more than men in the over 45 age group but more men than women under that age. Commonly referred to as the 'wear and tear' disease, osteoarthritis is the result of degeneration of tissue and the growth of bony spurs (osteophytes) in a joint which causes stiffness, pain and sometimes swelling. If left untreated the joint can become deformed and lose all function.

Osteoarthritis can occur in any synovial joint, usually a weight-bearing joint such as the knee, hip, lower back and neck, but can also be a problem in the shoulders, thumbs, fingers and big toes.

- *Hips*: Mainly affects men and women after middle age and can be quite severe requiring hip replacement surgery.
- *Knees*: Can be caused by being overweight; through continual mechanical stress on the joint; or injury through accident or sport.
- *Hands*: Commonly found in women, especially if there is a family history of osteoarthritis. Areas most affected are the fingertip joints and the base of the thumb.
- *Spine*: The neck and the lower back are the most common sites for osteoarthritis (spondylitis). In this instance there is also wearing of the discs between the spinal vertebrae.

Symptoms

These can vary from person to person. Some people may experience only mild or occasional pain in their joint/s, while others may suffer stiffness, swelling and severe pain which persists even when they're resting.

- *Hip*: Pain may be felt in the groin or the front of the thigh when walking or standing for any length of time. In some cases it persists when the person is resting too. Stiffness can make the sufferer reluctant to walk or exercise, inactivity adds to the stiffness, which in turn leads to immobility.
- *Knees*: There may be stiffness in the knee after sitting or standing for long periods, plus pain and swelling. The muscles and ligaments supporting the knee can become weak from lack of exercise, and you may feel that the whole joint has become unstable.
- *Hands*: Intermittent pain, swelling and redness. If the osteoarthritis is in the base of the thumb, then gripping or holding actions may become painful and difficult.
- *Spine*: When the neck is affected it can lead to stiffness, decreased range of motion and pain which may also be 'referred' down the arm. If osteoarthritis is present in the lower back, then there may be stiffness when rising from a seated or lying position, or pain when standing or sitting for any length of time; there may also be 'referred' pain down the legs.

Cause

It is thought to result from cellular changes within the joint which cause the cartilage to thin, become brittle, develop splits and flake off. As a result the joint becomes stiff, swollen and painful. As the condition persists the cartilage becomes so eroded that raw bone is exposed. Over time osteophytes grow out from the margins of the bone causing more injury to the joint and finally deformity, which is particularly noticeable and disabling in the hands.

In younger people osteoarthritis can be caused by:

An osteoarthritic joint

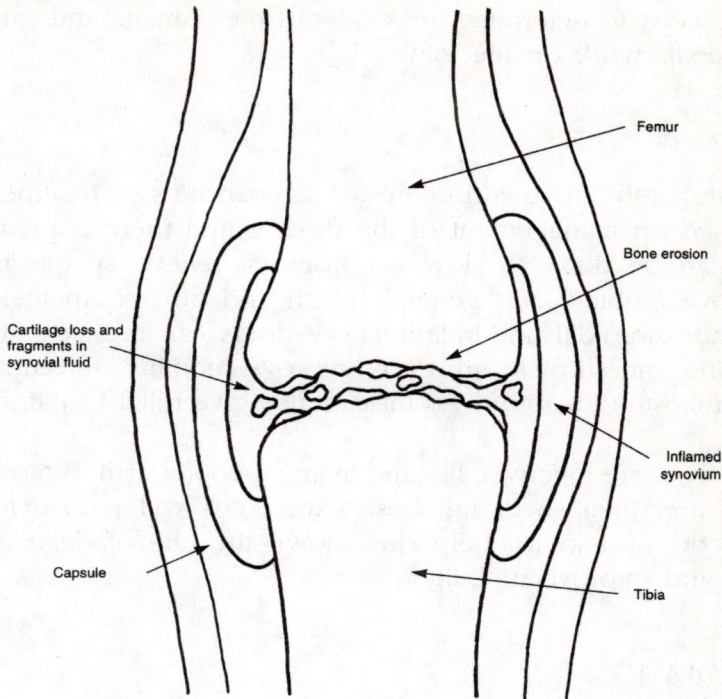

- Femur
- Bone erosion
- Cartilage loss and fragments in synovial fluid
- Inflamed synovium
- Capsule
- Tibia

- congenital deformities which result in mechanical malfunction of a joint
- a slight misalignment of the bones which causes uneven wear
- excessive injury through sport.

Many footballers, joggers and basketball players suffer from osteoarthritis from their middle years due to cartilage damage in their knees during their playing days.

Diagnosis

Osteoarthritis is usually diagnosed from symptoms and x-rays which can confirm the presence of osteophytes, cartilage, joint or bone damage. If these prove inconclusive your doctor may order blood tests or analysis of fluid from the joint to rule out other forms of arthritis. If osteoarthritis is suspected in the knee, it may be recommended that you have an arthroscopy to determine the extent of the damage and carry out repair work on the joint.

Treatment

Unfortunately, there is no cure for osteoarthritis so treatment is based on management of the disease and there is plenty that can be done to slow its progress, relieve symptoms, improve mobility and general health and fitness. Analgesic and non-steroidal anti-inflammatory drugs can reduce pain, swelling and stiffness and thus improve mobility. Injections of corticosteroids into the joint can also give relief to painful joints.

If you are overweight, and many people with osteoarthritis are, then shedding those extra kilos will reduce the stress on your joints, help slow down the rate of degeneration and improve mobility.

OSTEOPATHY

Osteopathy is a complementary medicine which not only takes into consideration physical symptoms but also a patient's lifestyle, attitudes and current health status.

Osteopaths believe that the human body has an ability to heal itself and that poor health and disease can result from a problem with the musculo-skeletal structure of the body. They are trained to recognise, diagnose and treat disorders of the musculo-skeletal system, and related areas such as ligaments and tendons, including arthritis, back and neck problems, joint pain, migraine and tension headaches among other things.

OSTEOPHYTES

Usually seen in osteoarthritis, these are bony spurs which grow out from the margins of bones in a joint, often occurring due to degeneration of cartilage or discs.

OSTEOTOMY

This is an operation in which a bone is cut and repositioned to change its alignment, or lengthen or shorten it. Realigning a bone is sometimes required to correct a deformity which causes undue wear and tear in a joint. If performed on the tibia, for example, this operation not only relieves pain but can often stop or reverse the damage caused by osteoarthritis of the knee.

PHYSIOTHERAPY

Physiotherapy is the treatment of diseases, disorders or injuries by physical methods. A physiotherapist can use a broad range of treatments which successfully reduce pain for arthritis sufferers, increase joint flexibility, reduce swelling and inflammation and advise on appropriate exercise programs. Treatments can include ultrasound and electrical stimulation such as TENS (transcutaneous electric nerve stimulation) and diathermy, which are used in addition to a program of massage, joint mobilisation and posture correction.

PROBENICID

Probenicid (Benemid) is a uricosuric drug used in the treatment of gout to reduce the level of uric acid in the blood stream. If taking this drug, you should be carefully monitored as it can cause allergic reactions or gastrointestinal upsets in some people.

PSORIATIC ARTHRITIS

This is inflammation of the joints in people who suffer from psoriasis (or who eventually develop psoriasis). It occurs in about one in 10 patients with this skin disease, which is characterised by areas of thickened, inflamed, often scaly, skin. The cause of psoriasis is unknown but it does seem to be hereditary. Although mostly likely to appear between the ages of 10 and 30 years of age, it can also occur in young children and older people. Psoriatic arthritis is treated in a similar way to rheumatoid arthritis with NSAIDs, sulphasalazine, methotrexate and corticosteroids.

QUERCETIN

Pronounced kwer-se-tin, this is a chemical found in plant foods which has been shown to have powerful antioxidant and anti-inflammatory actions on the body, as well as being a mild sedative—all properties which are beneficial to arthritis sufferers, especially those with autoimmune disorders, such as rheumatoid arthritis and SLE. Major sources of quercetin are red and brown onions, shallots, red grapes, broccoli and yellow button squash.

REMISSION

This is when symptoms of a disease temporarily and unexpectedly disappear or reduce significantly for a period of time, which can be anywhere from a few weeks to several years. Some forms of arthritis, such as rheumatoid arthritis, are subject to remissions.

RESECTION

This is the removal of some or all of a bone, and is often performed when a damaged joint or bunion in the foot causes problems with walking. It is also sometimes performed to reduce pain and improve function in the elbow, wrist or thumb.

RHEUMATOID ARTHRITIS

Rheumatoid arthritis is an autoimmune disease which causes pain, stiffness and swelling in one or more joints. Unlike osteoarthritis, rheumatoid arthritis occurs in previously normal joints and is triggered by some unknown factor. Onset can be sudden or gradual, confined to a single bout, or experienced as a prolonged series of attacks.

A joint affected by rheumatoid arthritis

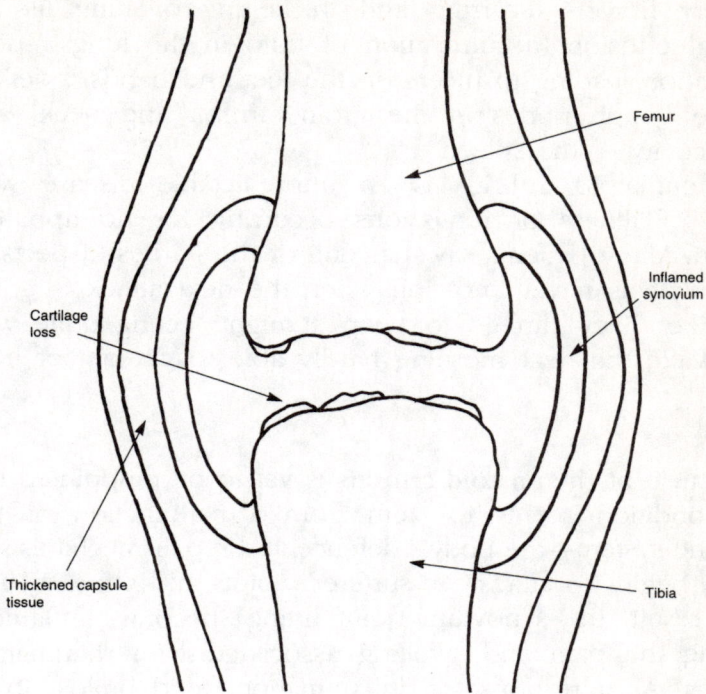

Symptoms

These can also vary from person to person with some patients experiencing only minor aches and pains, while others are totally debilitated by the disease. Symptoms include:

- mild fever
- aches and pain in and around a joint (joints on both sides of the body are usually equally affected)
- joint stiffness, particularly in the morning
- swollen joints, especially the feet, knees and hands
- a constant feeling of being tired and run down
- weakness in the muscles, ligaments and tendons surrounding the joint
- sleeplessness caused by pain and an inability to find a comfortable position.

In severe cases, complications can arise such as pericarditis

161

(inflammation of the membrane surrounding the heart), pulmonary fibrosis (scarring and thickening of lung tissue), pleural effusion (accumulation of fluid in the lungs), poor circulation leading to ulcers on the feet and hands, swelling of the lymph nodes in the groin, armpit and neck, and overactivity of the spleen.

Rheumatoid arthritis is an unpredictable disease with bouts of illness or remissions occurring for no apparent reason. Many patients say that one of the hardest aspects to cope with is never knowing when the next attack is going to strike. They can go to sleep at night feeling quite well and wake the next morning hardly able to get out of bed.

Cause

The cause of rheumatoid arthritis is yet to be pinpointed but the condition seems to stem from a malfunction of the immune system—the body's defence and repair mechanism—which begins to attack the sufferer's joints and other tissues. As a result, the synovium (joint lining) becomes inflamed, causing the pain and swelling associated with rheumatoid arthritis. As a response to inflammation, fluid builds up in the joint and the cells and other inflammatory products produced by the synovium attack the cartilage, cause weakening of the joint capsule and erosions in the bone itself. A vicious cycle of attack and defence is set up and, if left untreated, the whole system of the joint breaks down.

Although rheumatoid arthritis can occur in any joint it most commonly affects those of the fingers, wrists, shoulders, knees, hips and neck.

Onset of this disease usually starts in early adulthood but it can also develop in children. Women are three times more likely to suffer from this disease than men and, sadly, it often strikes them in their thirties just at a time when their career or family responsibilities are at their greatest.

Diagnosis

This is usually made from the patient's symptoms and medical history, blood tests (to identify an antibody called rheumatoid factor), and x-rays of the joint/s which helps determine whether damage to bones or cartilage has occurred. Sometimes a test called erythrocyte sedimentation rate (ESR) is performed to assess the degree of disease activity. A high ESR means the disease is very active.

Treatment

There is no cure for rheumatoid arthritis, however, effective treatment can manage the disease and will ensure that quality of life can be maintained with less pain and fewer physical disabilities. While analgesics and non-steroidal anti-inflammatory drugs can provide some symptom relief, the main medications used in the treatment of rheumatoid arthritis are the disease-modifying anti-rheumatic drugs. Medications include:

- analgesics
- non-steroidal anti-inflammatory drugs
- anti-rheumatic drugs
- anti-malarial drugs
- corticosteroids
- D-penicillamine
- gold salts
- immunosuppressant drugs
- sulphasalazine.

Physiotherapy, hydrotherapy, occupational therapy, surgery and education classes can also significantly help in the management of rheumatoid arthritis.

RHEUMATOID FACTOR

This is an antibody produced by the immune system in patients suffering from rheumatoid arthritis.

SERONEGATIVE ARTHRITIS

A number of conditions come under this name, all of which mimic the symptoms of rheumatoid arthritis in a number of joints, but show up as negative when blood tests are taken for the disease. Seronegative arthritis can be associated with Crohn's disease, which is an inflammatory disorder of the intestines, autoimmune disorders, and skin conditions such as psoriasis. Treatment is similar to that for rheumatoid arthritis.

SOFT TISSUE RELEASE

This is a procedure which involves surgically releasing contracted tendons, ligaments and other soft tissue in severe cases of rheumatoid arthritis.

SULFINPYRAZONE

Sulfinpyrazone (Auturan) is a uricosuric drug used to treat gout by increasing the ability of the kidneys to excrete uric acid from the blood stream.

SULPHASALAZINE (SALAZOPYRIN EN)

One of the stronger drugs used in the treatment of rheumatoid arthritis and psoriatic arthritis, sulphasalazine reduces inflammation and prevents flare-ups, thus helping to limit damage to joints. A few people do experience nausea, indigestion, dizziness and headache in the first three months of taking this drug, which can usually be eased by adjusting the prescription. If, however, you develop severe mouth ulcers, sore throats or excessive bruising, stop taking the medication immediately and consult your doctor. Another temporary side effect in men is a reduced sperm count which reverts to normal on stopping the drug.

SURGERY

If medical treatment is no longer easing your symptoms and your quality of life is being affected, then it may be time to consider surgery to restore mobility and relieve your pain. Surgical options include arthrodesis (fusion of the bones), arthroplasty (joint reconstruction), arthroscopy (examination and repair of a joint), osteotomy (realignment of the bones), resection (removal of some or all of the bone), synovectomy (removal of diseased synovium), tendon repair and soft tissue release.

Today, surgical techniques can repair tendons and ligaments damaged by disease, extend the life of a diseased joint or replace it if it has degenerated to the point where it no longer functions. It's amazing the number of people for whom corrective or replacement surgery has given a new lease on life and over the last decade or so tremendous advances have been made in this area. Lighter, more durable materials have allowed prostheses to be produced where the bone actually grows through the device, locking it into place. Combined with better operating techniques and after-surgery care, this has meant that joint replacement now has an extremely high success rate.

Having said that, however, surgery is not something you should go into without careful thought. There are some risks, as there are with any surgery, and to achieve a successful outcome will take hard work and commitment on your part. So, it's important that you understand all aspects of any surgery that is recommended—the procedures and implications involved—before you go ahead with an operation.

Firstly find out as much as you can about the proposed operation and ask your doctor the following questions:

- Is there any other non-surgical treatment which could help you?
- How successful is the operation?
- What outcome should you expect?
- How will it improve your quality of life?
- What will happen if you don't have the operation?
- What risks are involved?
- What if the operation isn't successful?
- What does the procedure involve?
- How long will you be in hospital?
- How long before you are up and about again?
- What after-care/treatment will be required?
- How long before you are totally recovered from this operation?

- And, if you have private health insurance, what will it cost and how much will you be out of pocket?

You will also have to answer some questions for yourself:

- Can you afford the time off work, especially if you are self-employed?
- Do you have someone who can take over your family responsibilities for the time you are in hospital and during the recovery period?
- Are you prepared to accept the pain and discomfort which might be involved in such an operation?
- Are you prepared to commit yourself to the rehabilitation program?
- And for those of you with private health insurance, can you afford the gap between what the operation and after-care services will cost and what you will be refunded by your health insurance company?

Once these questions have been answered you'll be in a position to decide whether or not you are prepared to go ahead with the operation.

Prior to the operation

If you have other health problems, such as obesity, hypertension (high blood pressure), heart or lung disease, these will have to be under control before you can have any operation. For example, if you are overweight, you should lose those extra kilos to lessen the stress not only on your joints but also on your heart and lungs. If you have hypertension (high blood pressure), this should be well under control through appropriate medication, adopting a low-salt diet and losing weight if you are over your weight-for-height range. Prior to surgery you will also have to be free of any bacterial infection as it could spread through your blood stream to the operative site.

How surgery can help you

- *Hands*: Loss of function in your hands is both physically

Knee replacement

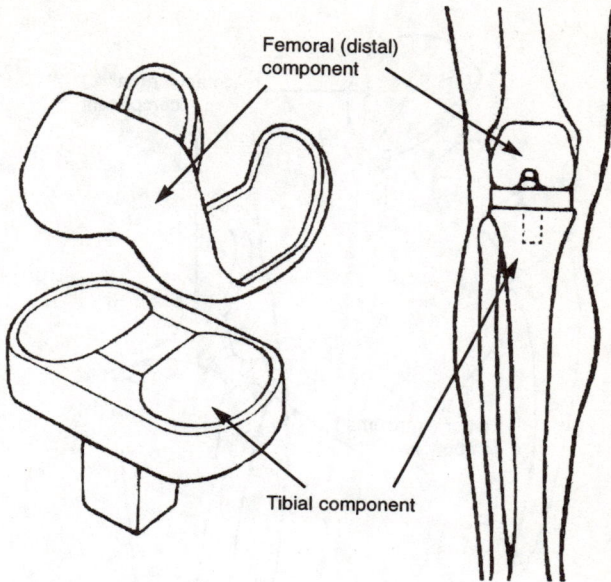

Femoral (distal) component

Tibial component

and mentally disabling. It can make simple tasks such as eating, washing or dressing very difficult which creates a sense of frustration and helplessness in arthritis sufferers. Surgery can not only reduce pain and restore function, it can also correct deformity, which can have a positive psychological benefit. There are several operations which can be performed on the hand—synovectomy to relieve pain and prevent fingers becoming deformed; tendon repair to improve function; joint replacement to relieve pain, restore function and correct deformity; and arthrodesis to stop pain and prevent further damage to the joint.

- *Wrists*: Arthritis in the wrists can cause a great deal of pain and loss of function in the hands. Fortunately, there are several procedures which can help, including arthrodesis, which although it will stiffen the wrist is extremely effective in relieving pain and stabilising other joints in the hand.
- *Knee*: Arthroscopy is one of the most common operations

Hip replacement

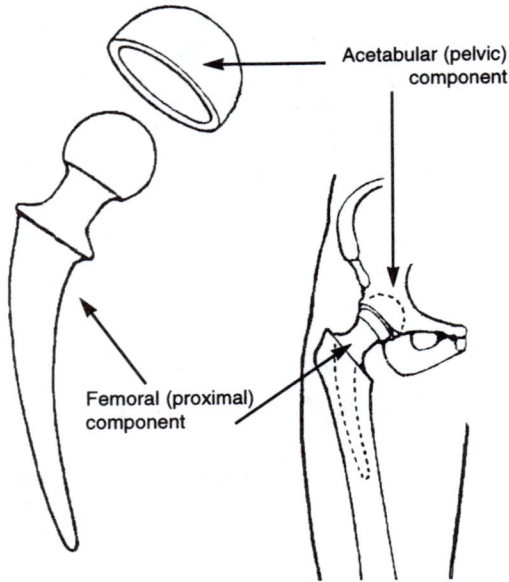

Acetabular (pelvic)
component

Femoral (proximal)
component

performed on the knee. It is done to assess the condition of the joint, to remove loose material or fluid, carry out repair work on torn cartilage and ligaments, and smooth the surface of the kneecap.

Synovectomy, to remove a diseased synovium, can prevent the inflammation and pain caused by severe rheumatoid arthritis.

Osteotomy is performed to stop or reverse the damage caused by osteoarthritis. This operation involves cutting and repositioning the tibia to change its alignment to prevent undue wear and tear in the knee joint.

Total knee replacement (see figure on previous page) is commonly performed on people over the age of 60, whose knees have been damaged by osteo- or rheumatoid arthritis. In this operation the surfaces of the upper end of the shin bone (tibia) and the lower end of the thigh bone (femur) are cut away and the bone drilled and shaped to accept a prosthesis, made of metal and polyethylene, which is then screwed and/or cemented in place. A cast is usually placed over the knee after the operation and kept on for about five days, after which time a program of exercises is required to strengthen the quadriceps muscles. It takes two to three weeks before you're able to put weight on the leg, and full recovery can take several months.

- *Hip*: The most common operation on the hip is joint replacement (see figure on previous page). In this operation the ball and socket joint in the hip is replaced by a prosthesis. The top of the thigh bone (femur) is removed, a shaft cut into it and the ball component inserted. A hollow is then drilled into the pelvis and a cup-shaped socket is inserted. The ball is then placed into the socket and the hip reconstructed. As the joint remains unstable for one or two weeks after the operation great care must be taken not to dislocate the hip. Full recovery can take several months.
- *Foot and ankle*: When arthritis affects the feet it makes walking extremely difficult and painful. Several operations can be performed to relieve pain and restore function, including synovectomy, resection, tendon repair and replacement surgery. However, the mechanical structure of the ankle and foot is extremely complex so careful evaluation should be undertaken before any operation is performed.

Recovery

It's important, with any of these operations, to adopt a positive mental attitude. Not only will it reduce your mental stress but it will go a long way toward achieving a successful physical outcome. You will also have to make a commitment to follow post-operative treatment such as rest, physical therapy and limiting activity to ensure a full and speedy recovery. This may mean taking things easy for a while, and using a walking stick or crutches. You will probably be given a series of exercises to perform and told not to put too much weight on the joint. How well you follow this advice can make all the difference to the success of the operation.

You may also have to learn how to do some things differently. For example, if you have had a hip replacement, you may need to alter some positions used for love making, or avoid certain exercises in aqua- or hydrotherapy classes; if you have had knee surgery, kneeling while cleaning the house or gardening may be prohibited. It's important to follow your doctor's advice to prevent set backs. A physio- or occupational therapist will also be able to give you information on the best way to do things.

If you follow doctor's orders, stick to your exercise routine, rest, and avoid any inappropriate activity, you will find you have a whole new lifestyle to look forward to!

SYNOVECTOMY

This operation, to remove a diseased synovium, is only performed after all drug therapy has failed to prevent the inflammation and pain caused by severe rheumatoid arthritis. The procedure involves the removal of the synovial membrane lining a joint or tendon sheath to prevent or slow down destructive synovitis. It should be noted, however, that the synovium can grow back over time and the problems recur.

SYNOVIUM

This is a membrane lining the joint capsule which produces fluid to lubricate the joint, nourish the cartilage, and remove any waste products from the area.

SYSTEMIC LUPUS ERYTHEMATOSUS (SLE)

Systemic lupus erythematosus (SLE) is a chronic inflammatory disease affecting many parts of the body. It's commonly known as lupus. Like rheumatoid arthritis, SLE is an auto-immune disease which causes inflammation and damage to joints, other body tissues and organs. It is subject to flare-ups and remissions like other inflammatory arthritis and is treated in much the same way as rheumatoid arthritis. SLE affects more women than men, usually between the ages of 18 and 45 years, however it can occur in children and older people.

Symptoms

Although symptoms vary from person to person they can include fever, weakness, fatigue, weight loss, rashes on the face, neck and arms and sometimes the nose and cheeks (frequently referred to as the 'butterfly rash' of SLE); there may also be morning stiffness and joint pain in the hands, wrists, elbows, knees or ankles; muscles aches, swollen glands, loss of appetite, hair loss, nausea and vomiting may also be experienced. These symptoms can be precipitated or worsened by exposure to sunlight. Occasionally, an SLE patient may suffer from Raynaud's syndrome, which is unusual sensitivity to cold in the hands and fingers. Because their immune system is compromised, SLE patients are prone to infections, and may develop anaemia and an increased tendency to form blood clots. Other less obvious symptoms can include inflammation of the linings in the heart and lungs, and kidney problems.

Cause

As yet no-one knows what causes SLE and there is no known cure. Some studies suggest that there may be an hereditary link to this disease, while others point to a virus being the trigger for its onset, however, the jury is still out and further research is needed to identify its true cause.

Diagnosis

This is made from the signs and symptoms such as the 'butterfly rash' and sensitivity to sunlight, blood tests, urine analysis, and chest x-rays to determine whether the heart and lungs have been affected.

Treatment

Treatment is similar to that for rheumatoid arthritis, consisting of medication to reduce inflammation and autoimmune activity in the body, resting when the disease is active, and close monitoring of health. As different treatment suits different people, it's important that time is taken to find the right treatment for you. It may take several weeks or months of trial and error with medications to find which ones work best for you. Medications include non-steroidal anti-inflammatory drugs (NSAIDs), anti-malarial drugs, corticosteroids, and immunosuppressive drugs. SLE is an unpredictable disease, which varies from person to person and can flare-up or go into remission for no apparent reason.

TAI CHI

This is an ancient Chinese ritual of movements designed to promote health and well-being throughout the body. All Tai Chi movements work to release tension, mobilise stiff joints, improve circulation and reduce stress. In Tai Chi, joints are taken through a slow, gentle range of movements and stiff joints are not made to move more than they are able. Tai Chi exercises also avoid sudden changes in direction and movements are absorbed by the muscles rather than the joints. These smooth flowing, relaxed exercises allow increased blood supply to flow to the joints, improving their function and condition. Many people suffering from arthritis who have taken up Tai Chi have found it has reduced their pain and stress levels, given them greater flexibility, increased muscle tone and improved their outlook on life. Many Tai Chi instructors these days run classes especially designed for arthritis sufferers.

TENDON REPAIR

A patient with long-term active rheumatoid arthritis can develop contracted tendons, which not only restrict movements but cause severe pain. Sometimes performed along with other surgical procedures, this operation involves releasing tight tendons, ligaments and other soft tissue structures. Sometimes tendons become too loose and an operation will be performed to tighten them.

TENS

A transcutaneous electric nerve stimulation (TENS) machine is an electronic device used to relieve pain. It works by stimulating various nerve pathways to the brain, which encourages the body to release endorphins.

THALAMUS

This is a mass of nerve tissue that sits at the top of the brain stem. Shaped like two eggs but the size of a walnut, the thalamus is connected to all parts of the brain and is an important relay centre for sensory information from the eyes, ears and the spinal cord. It is through the thalamus that pain is relayed to the brain.

ULTRASOUND

In this treatment, high-frequency sound waves are used to promote blood flow through soft tissue, thereby reducing inflammation and speeding up the healing process.

VEGETARIANISM

There has been much debate about the role of diet in diseases such as rheumatoid arthritis and while many doctors pooh-pooh the idea that food can influence the nature of this illness, there are some studies which show that adopting a vegetarian diet seems to improve symptoms for some patients. In 1991, Norwegian doctors at the Institute of Immunology at the National Rheumatology Hospital in Oslo discovered that switching to a vegan vegetarian diet reduced the symptoms of pain, swelling and morning stiffness in nine out of ten patients with rheumatoid arthritis.

XUAN SHEN

This is a Chinese herb, similar to the Western herb figwort, which has been used to treat rheumatism and gout for hundreds of years in the East. The flowers and aerial parts (leaves and stems, in fact all parts above the ground except the flowers) are used to make infusions and tinctures, and a compress can be made using a warm tea made from the dried herb. It is best to consult a qualified Chinese herbalist if you wish to try this herb as it is not suitable for all people, especially not those with heart problems.

YUCCA

This is a herb traditionally used by both North and South American Indians for the relief of arthritic pain. Taken either as a tea or in tablet form, herbalists claim that it can bring relief in as little as three days, but may take up to three months to show beneficial results. Some scientific studies are taking place of its usefulness as an arthritis cure. The jury is still out on this one.

ZINGIBER OFFICINALE (GINGER)

Long thought by the Chinese to bring relief to arthritis patients, studies in Germany have now shown ginger to contain anti-inflammatory substances which can reduce pain, swelling, stiffness and mobility. Used in cooking, or taken as a tea or tablet, ginger may be a useful addition to arthritis therapy.

Where to go for help and further information

ARTHRITIS FOUNDATION CENTRES

Arthritis Foundation of Australia
Suite 902A, Kindersley House,
33 Bligh Street,
Sydney,
NSW 2000
Telephone: (02) 9221 2456
Fax: (02) 9232 2538

New South Wales

Arthritis Foundation of NSW
69–75 Reservoir Street,
Surry Hills,
NSW 2010
Telephone: (02) 9281 1611
Fax: (02) 9281 4473

Australian Capital Territory

Arthritis Foundation of ACT
Health Promotion Centre,
Childers Street,

Canberra City,
ACT 2600
Telephone: (02) 6257 4842
Fax: (02) 6249 6999

Victoria

Arthritis Foundation of Victoria
263–265 Kooyong Road,
Elsternwick,
Victoria 3185
Telephone   (03) 9530 0255
Fax: (03) 9530 0220

Queensland

Arthritis Foundation of Queensland
QEII Jubilee Hospital, Kessels Road,
Coopers Plains,
Queensland 4108
Telephone   (07) 3274 1360
Fax: (07) 3274 1363

South Australia

Arthritis Foundation of South Australia
99 Anzac Highway,
Ashford,
South Australia 5035
Telephone: (08) 8297 2488
Fax: (08) 8293 1177

Western Australia

Arthritis Foundation of Western Australia
17 Lemnos Street,
Shenton Park,
Western Australia 6008
Telephone: (08) 9388 2199
Fax: (08) 9388 4488

Tasmania

Arthritis Foundation of Tasmania
30/84 Hampden Road,
Battery Point,
Tasmania 7004
Telephone: (03) 2346 489
Fax: (03) 2346 489

Northern Territory

Arthritis Foundation of Northern Territory
PO Box 37582
Winnellie,
Northern Territory 0822
Telephone: (08) 9832 071
Fax: (08) 9832 449

New Zealand

Arthritis Foundation of New Zealand
159 Featherstone Street,
Wellington,
New Zealand
Telephone: NZ (4) 721 427
Fax: NZ (4) 723 967

INDEPENDENT LIVING CENTRES

New South Wales

600 Victoria Road,
Ryde, NSW 2112,
Telephone: (02) 9808 2233, 1800 800 523
Info Line: (02) 9808 2477
Fax: (02) 9809 7132

Australian Capital Territory

24 Parkinson Street,
Weston, ACT 2611

Telephone: (02) 6205 1900
Fax: (02) 6205 1906

Victoria

52 Thistlethwaite Street,
South Melbourne, Victoria 3205
Telephone: (03) 9254 5400
Fax: (03) 9696 1956

Queensland

388 Cavendish Road,
Coorparoo, Queensland 4151
Telephone: (07) 3397 1224
Fax: (07) 3394 1013

South Australia

180 Daws Road,
Daw Park, South Australia 5041
Telephone: (08) 8276 3455, 1800 800 523
Fax: (08) 8276 7417

Western Australia

3 Lemnos Street,
Shenton Park,
Western Australia 6008
Telephone: (08) 9382 2011, 1800 800 523
Fax: (08) 9382 2896

Tasmania

46 Canning Street,
Launceston, Tasmania 7250
Telephone: (03) 2345 899
Fax: (03) 2340 045

Index